KW-482-513

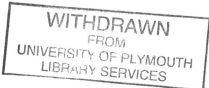

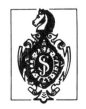

Neil B. Solomons

Practical Introduction to ENT Disease

With 19 Figures

Springer-Verlag
London Berlin Heidelberg New York
Paris Tokyo Hong Kong

Neil B. Solomons, FRCS
Senior Registrar in Otolaryngology, Royal Free Hospital,
Pond Street, London NW3 2QG and Royal Surrey County
Hospital, Egerton Road, Guildford, Surrey GU2 5XX, UK

ISBN 3-540-19566-1 Springer-Verlag Berlin Heidelberg New York
ISBN 0-387-19566-1 Springer-Verlag New York Berlin Heidelberg

British Library Cataloguing in Publication Data
Solomons, Neil B. *1955–*
    Practical introduction to ENT disease.
    1. Man. Ears, nose & throat. Diseases & injuries
    I. Title   617'.51
    ISBN 3–540–19566–1

Library of Congress Cataloging-in-Publication Data
Solomons, Neil B., 1955–
    Practical introduction to ENT disease/Neil B. Solomons
    p. cm.   Includes bibliographical references
    ISBN 0–387–19566–1
    1. Otolaryngology. 2. Family medicine. I. Title
    [DNLM: 1. Otorhinolaryngologic Diseases—therapy. WV 100 S689p]
RF46.5.S65   1989   617.5'1—dc20
DNLM/DLC
for Library of Congress   89-21628
                                                           CIP

Typeset by Macmillan India Ltd., Bangalore 560 025
Printed by The Bath Press, Avon

2128/3916-543210   Printed on acid-free paper

Preface

Why an ENT book specifically for those in General Practice?

The time devoted to ENT in the undergraduate curriculum is rather limited when contrasted with the ENT content of a General Practitioner's work. Only a small minority of intending General Practitioners will do a post-registration ENT job. The majority of ENT textbooks presently available are aimed at imparting basic information to medical students or are written for those pursuing a career in ENT. An analysis of patient referrals to ENT departments in Gloucestershire, along with the results of questionnaires used at the annual ENT course for GPs held in Gloucester, realised the need for this book.

The book is problem-orientated, practical and, it is hoped, provides a useful guide of when to refer, when to treat and how to treat. Detailed anatomy and physiology are covered in the standard texts and are therefore not included here. References are purposefully excluded but content reflects current thinking in the world of otolaryngology. There will obviously be areas of controversy but the views expressed are those commonly held by the majority of my colleagues. The emphasis is on daily practical problems and deliberately avoids detail of conditions a GP may only see once or twice in a lifetime of practice.

I sincerely hope this book is not only useful to GPs in their handling of everyday ENT problems, but that it also furthers a harmonious relationship between the General Practitioner in the community and the specialist in the hospital.

I am most grateful to Jeremy Barnes, a senior Gloucester GP, for his advice and input from the General Practitioner's point of view. I am particularly indebted to all my teachers for their advice and training.

To those who lent secretarial assistance and word-processing advice, in particular Jane Polley, I offer my sincere thanks.

Finally, to my wife and children I express a deep sense of appreciation for tolerating my obsession with "the book"!

Surrey, February 1989   Neil B. Solomons

Contents

1 The ENT Examination

Any patient complaining of a symptom relating to the ENT system should have that entire system examined. The same principle would apply to the cardiovascular or respiratory systems and the ENT system is therefore not exceptional. An adequate history obviously precedes this examination. The doctor should be seated facing the patient, who is also sitting. A good light source is mandatory. The practitioner can use a head mirror with an appropriate light source (e.g. anglepoise lamp, Welch–Allen lamp) or a head light can be worn. Both these methods not only provide a good source of light but they also allow the freedom to use both hands to examine the patient. A head mirror requires some practice to focus the light in the appropriate place but the use of a head light is considerably easier.

As ENT problems feature prominently in everyday General Practice, it is necessary to have the essential basic instruments to examine these patients. Exmoor Plastics supply a very good "minimum requirements" pack and the recommended instruments are shown in Fig. 1.1.

The various components of the examination may be performed in any order but the practitioner should develop an ordered routine which is followed on all patients. The following is a useful guide. Commence by examining the oral cavity. This should include a good inspection of the lips, buccal mucosa, the gums and teeth (patients with dentures should remove these prior to examination), the tongue, tonsils (if still present), the posterior pharyngeal wall and the hard and soft palates. It is a good idea at this stage to ask the patient to say "aaah" as this will allow the assessment of palatal mobility (cranial nerves: sensory IX, motor X). The tongue should be protruded not only to permit inspection of a greater part of its surface but also to assess the function of the hypoglossal nerve (XIIth cranial nerve). If any area of the buccal cavity gives cause for doubt or concern, the area should be palpated as this often gives the examiner a better idea of a lesion than visual inspection alone. The buccal mucosa, the floor of the mouth and the submandibular and parotid salivary glands should be palpated bimanually (Fig. 1.2). Intra-oral palpation should always be performed using a gloved finger, as this will minimise the risks of transmissible diseases. This is particularly important where there is great concern about the AIDS virus.

The next area of examination is the nose. First the external appearance should be noted. In children, a reasonable view of the anterior part of the

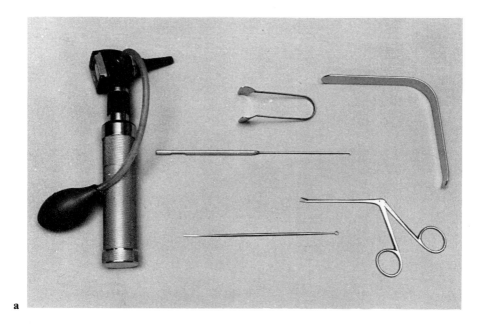

a

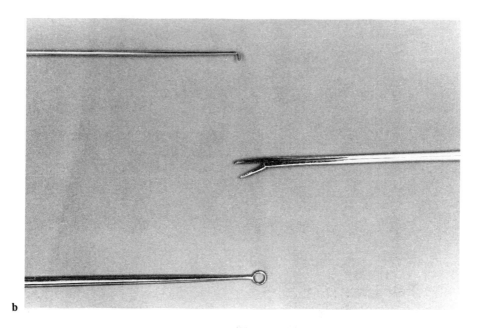

b

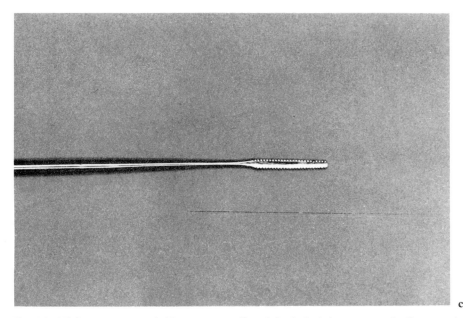

c

Fig. 1.1. Minimum recommended instruments. **a** (from left, clockwise) auroscope, thudicum nasal speculum, tongue depressor, crocodile forceps, Jobson–Horne probe (ring probe) and (centre) wax hook. **b** Detail of (top to bottom) wax hook, crocodile forceps and Jobson–Horne probe (ring end). **c** Serrated end of Jobson–Horne probe.

septum and inferior turbinates can be obtained merely by elevating the nasal tip (Fig. 1.3). In adults the firmer cartilaginous structure of the nasal tip makes this method of examination less satisfactory and instrumentation is therefore often necessary. A nasal speculum is gently inserted into each nostril in turn. As the blades of the speculum are parted inspection of the intranasal anatomy becomes possible (Fig. 1.4). This is known as anterior rhinoscopy. The nasal speculum should be of the right size. If the speculum is too large, the examination is difficult for the examiner and uncomfortable for the patient. If the speculum is too small, an inadequate view is obtained. Posterior rhinoscopy is performed using a post-nasal mirror, but this is not a skill expected of non-ENT surgeons.

When performing anterior rhinoscopy, deviations of the septum should be noted, the size and colour of the inferior turbinates should be documented and a search made for the presence of abnormal lesions (e.g. polyps). The appearances are dealt with in Chap. 4. Nasal airflow can be assessed crudely by observing the moisture on a mirror or silver spatula placed beneath the nose when the patient exhales nasally. Alternatively, one finger can occlude the undersurface of the opening of one nostril whilst the patient breathes through the other side (Fig. 1.5).

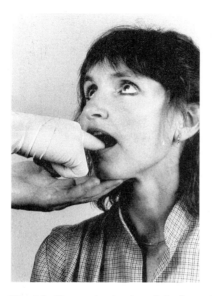

Fig. 1.2. Bimanual palpation of the floor of the mouth and submandibular salivary gland.

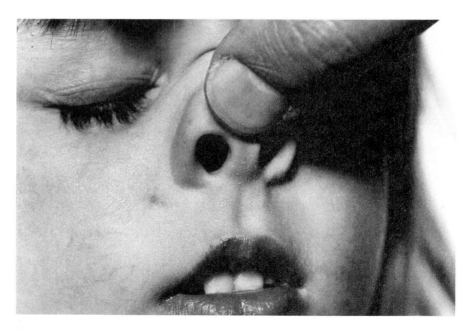

Fig. 1.3. Elevation of the nasal tip.

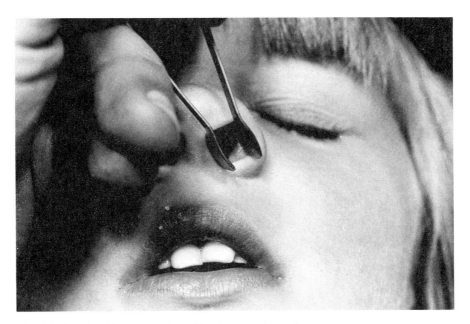

Fig. 1.4. Anterior rhinoscopy using a Thudicum nasal speculum.

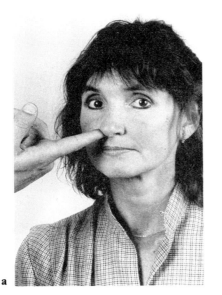
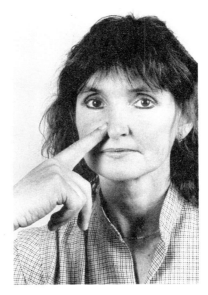

a

b

Fig. 1.5. Assessing nasal airflow. **a** Correct method. **b** Incorrect method. Compression of the alar surface of the nose may cause an artificial sensation of obstruction when the occluding finger is removed.

5

The ears are examined next. The appearance of the pinna is noted and the post-auricular area is examined for surgical scars before the auriscope is inserted into the external auditory meatus (EAM). If traction on the pinna causes pain, then pathology of the external canal should be suspected (see Chap. 2). An auriscope is then gently introduced into the EAM and should be held as shown in Fig. 1.6. Much is written of the direction in which to pull the pinna to permit visualisation of the tympanic membrane. However, there is no set rule about this and traction should be exerted in whichever direction facilitates straightening of the external canal.

The subject of wax is dealt with in Chap. 2. However, if wax is obscuring the view of the external canal and tympanic membrane, it should be removed if possible. This may be done using a Jobson–Horne probe (Fig. 1.1), a wax hook (Fig. 1.1), by syringing or using suction apparatus (as is often used in ENT clinics). It must be emphasised that the removal of wax should only be pursued as long as great difficulty is not encountered and as long as no discomfort is caused to the patient. Manual removal of wax requires good illumination to prevent any damage being caused to the external canal or tympanic membrane. If the wax is very hard it may be possible to soften it over a period of days by instilling sodium bicarbonate drops or olive oil into the affected ear. If difficulty persists, the patient should be referred for specialist assessment when the wax can be removed using a microscope and suction apparatus. If the task of removing wax is delegated to the practice nurse, she should be aware of the risks, the dangers and potential complications of such a procedure.

Proper use of the auriscope requires practice and "normal" ears should be carefully examined to appreciate the wide range of normality. An auriscope should always have an attached puffer (Fig. 1.7) so that the mobility of the

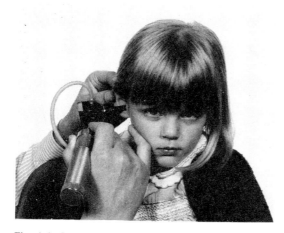

Fig. 1.6. Correct method of using the auroscope. Note the examiner's right hand guards against the patient's cheek in case sudden movement of the patient (children in particular) causes injury to the EAM.

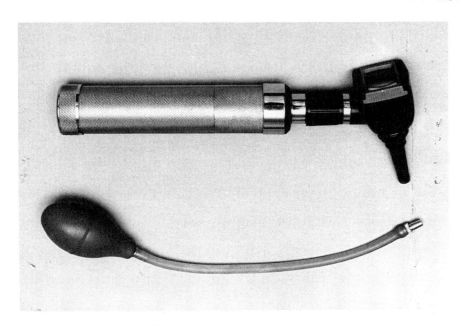

Fig. 1.7. Auroscope with puffer.

tympanic membrane can be assessed. The examiner should always use the biggest aural speculum possible (it is seldom necessary, even in infants, to use the smallest size speculum) to see as much of the anatomy as possible in one visual field. It is also preferable to use the longer variety of aural speculum (Fig. 1.8). The other important reason for using a big speculum is to obtain an air-tight seal when using the puffer.

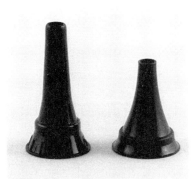

Fig. 1.8. Aural specula. It is preferable to use the longer variety of aural speculum.

When the speculum is inserted, the appearance of the canal wall should be noted. Otitis externa, a furuncle and exostoses should be seen if present at this stage. The tympanic mambrane may then be inspected and it is far from adequate to merely find (or not find!) the "light reflex". It is important to look at the attic, mesotympanum and hypotympanum in turn (Fig. 1.9). The malleus should then be inspected and in transparent drums the long process of the incus and incudo-stapedial joint can often be seen posterior to the malleus handle. It may indeed be possible to see erosion of this joint when the drum is markedly atrophic and retracted down onto it. Areas of retraction, especially retraction pockets and cholesteatoma, should actively be sought (see Chap. 2). The patient should then be warned of the impending puff of air when drum mobility is to be tested. The bulb of the puffer should be squeezed gently; the normal tympanic membrane will be seen to move medially then laterally when insufflated. There will be reduced or absent mobility if there is not an air-tight seal, but pathological reasons for impaired mobility include middle-ear effusion, marked tympanosclerosis (deposition of calcified plaques within the substance of the tympanic membrane) or the presence of a perforation. Atrophic areas or "healed perforations" can often resemble perforations but the diagnosis can be confirmed by insufflating the drum and observing the mobility of these areas. Occasionally the tympanic membrane has little "blebs" or scars on its surface which look like bubbles. An erroneous diagnosis of middle-ear fluid can be made in these cases but normal drum mobility should resolve this diagnostic problem.

The patient's hearing should then be assessed using tuning forks. The 512 Hz tuning fork is probably the most suitable for this purpose and the Weber and Rinne tests should be performed. These two tests will give the examining doctor a guide as to the type of hearing loss present and whether one or both ears are affected.

The Weber test is performed as follows (see Fig. 1.10). A vibrating tuning fork is placed in the midline of the patient's skull. This may be on the vertex, the

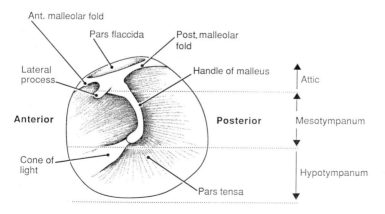

Fig. 1.9. Anatomy of the normal left tympanic membrane.

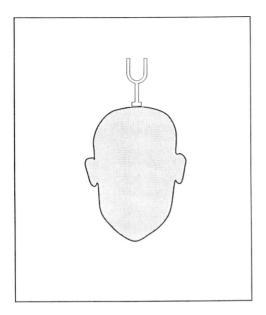

Fig. 1.10. Weber test

forehead, the nose or the teeth. The patient is then asked where the sound is heard. If it is heard in the midline, the hearing is either normal or any hearing loss is bilaterally symmetrical. If the sound is heard on one side, then either that ear has a significant (>25 db) conductive hearing loss or the other ear has a severe sensorineural hearing loss. The Rinne test will verify which of these two possibilities is more likely.

The Rinne test is performed as follows (see Fig. 1.11). A vibrating tuning fork is placed on the patient's mastoid process. When the patient reports that he no longer hears the vibration, the tuning fork is moved adjacent to the patient's EAM . If he now hears the sound, the Rinne test is said to be positive and there is no significant conductive hearing loss, i.e. the air conduction is better than bone conduction. The process is then repeated for the opposite ear. If the patient hears the sound better on the mastoid process, then the Rinne test is said to be negative, i.e. bone conduction is better than air conduction and this implies a significant conductive hearing loss (>25 db) on that side. There is one potential pitfall however if the test is negative. It may be possible that the "test" ear is in fact a non-hearing or "dead" ear. In this case, the reason that bone conduction indeed appears to be better is because the sound vibrations are being conducted through the skull bones to the opposite cochlea (the "good" ear). The results of tuning fork tests in malingerers may be confusing. If any doubt exists the patient should be referred to the local ENT department. The ENT surgeon and audiologist will usually be able to differentiate between organic and non-organic hearing loss (see Chap. 2, section on Non-organic Hearing Loss).

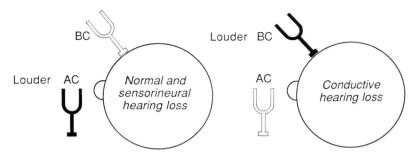

Fig. 1.11. Rinne test.

The ENT examination is not complete without examining the neck and temporo-mandibular joints. This is best done standing behind the seated patient. A random palpation of the neck in the hope that a mass will present itself under the examining fingers is unsatisfactory. A methodical palpation in a set pattern, e.g. submental triangle, submandibular regions, posterior and anterior triangles, is far more satisfactory. The thyroid gland should not be forgotten. The temporo-mandibular joints can then be palpated both with the mouth closed and with the mouth open. A significant number of patients who present with "earache" and who are referred to ENT clinics are found to have normal ears. Many of these patients' symptoms are due to temporo-mandibular joint dysfunction and it is wise to remember the areas from which otalgia may be referred (see Chap. 2). This is particularly relevant when there is no visible ear pathology.

2 The Ear

The Painful Ear

The patient complaining of a painful ear (otalgia) either has pathology in the ear or pain referred from some other site. The usual features of any pain should be sought, e.g. exact site, radiation, periodicity, aggravating and relieving factors etc. It is important to know whether there has been associated discharge from the ear (otorrhoea) and whether the patient has undergone ear surgery in the past. Details regarding recent swimming, air travel and the use of cotton buds should be elicited.

The examination of the patient with otalgia highlights the need for a complete examination of the head and neck as pain in the ear may be referred from so many other sites within that region. The ear has a diverse sensory innervation (Fig. 2.1) and disease processes causing otalgia may originate in any area having a similar sensory nerve supply. Pain in the ear may arise from pathology in the

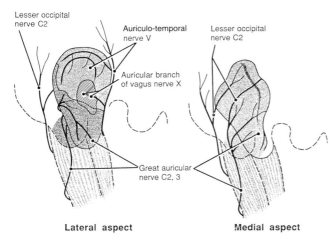

Fig. 2.1. Sensory innervation of the pinna and EAM. The middle-ear mucosa (including the medial aspect of the tympanic membrane) is supplied by the glossopharyngeal nerve (IX).

nose and paranasal sinuses, nasopharynx, teeth, jaws, temporo-mandibular joints, salivary glands and ducts, oropharynx, laryngopharynx, tongue and cervical spine. As mentioned in Chap. 1 , non-ENT surgeons are not expected to be proficient in the use of laryngeal and post-nasal mirrors, but failure to look in the mouth of a patient with otalgia could well be construed as an act of negligence. Although cancers of the tonsils and piriform fossa are not common (approximately 80 new tonsillar cancers per year in the UK), it is not unusual for such cancers to present with otalgia.

The aural causes of otalgia will now be discussed.

Diseases of the Pinna and External Auditory Meatus (EAM)

Otitis Externa

This is the commonest disorder of the EAM and occurs due to a variety of reasons or in association with several other conditions.

The patient with otitis externa will usually complain of pain in the ear, discharge from the ear and also a diminution in hearing if the EAM is swollen and filled with debris. Predisposing factors include eczema, seborrhoeic dermatitis of the scalp, diabetes (see necrotising otitis externa), psoriasis, swimming and cotton-bud abuse. Otitis externa is also more common in humid climates. Discharge of middle-ear fluid into the EAM may give rise to otitis externa but this is an infrequent association. It is not known why some patients can swim all year round with no ill-effects from constant wetting of the EAM skin whilst others will develop otitis externa following minimal exposure of the EAM to water. The use of cotton buds is a frequent association in patients with otitis externa seen in ENT clinics. This may be due to a hypersensitivity reaction or may result from trauma to the skin of the external canal if the cotton buds are used too vigorously.

Examination reveals tenderness on traction of the pinna. This is a feature of disorders of the EAM but is not a feature of middle-ear disease. There is often associated peri-auricular lymphadenopathy. The enlarged nodes may be pre-auricular, post-auricular and/or infra-auricular. In mild cases there is simply erythema of the EAM skin with some desquamation evident whilst in severe cases there is an abundance of desquamated debris surrounded by very tender, swollen canal walls. The entire meatus may be occluded by the swelling. If there is doubt as to whether an aural discharge arises from the middle ear or EAM, the presence or absence of mucus will indicate the origin of the discharge. There are no mucus-secreting glands in the EAM and the presence of mucus in the discharge usually implies a tympanic membrane perforation. The exception to the rule is granular myringitis (see below).

Management. The mainstay of treatment is aural toilet and the avoidance of any known or potential irritants (e.g. cotton buds, topical antibiotics). There is absolutely no point in pouring ear drops onto a bed of debris in the EAM. Gentle but thorough toilet is mandatory and if this cannot be carried out in the practitioner's surgery, the patient should be referred to an ENT surgeon who can then perform suction clearance of the EAM with the aid of an operating microscope. The degree of urgency of such a referral depends on the severity of the patient's symptoms. Syringing of the ears in the presence of any aural discharge is absolutely contraindicated. Once the debris has been cleared, appropriate ear drops can then be instilled into the EAM. The main action of such drops is to treat the inflammatory process rather than the "infection". There is little value in submitting bacteriological swabs from discharging ears as contaminants abound and the resident flora are more often cultured than not. Glycerine and ichthammol drops are extremely valuable in the treatment of this condition and the insertion of a "ribbon gauze" wick down the canal often facilitates the permeation of the drops right down to the tympanic membrane. Similarly, aluminium acetate (13%) can be used. When considerable oedema is present, small Merocel ear tampons may also be inserted into the canal. When the appropriate topical treatment is then applied, the tampon swells and thereby helps to open the canal. These are therefore only useful when the canal is occluded by oedema. The tampon should be removed after 48 hours. Steroid-containing drops (see Chap. 8) are also most valuable as they deal effectively with the inflammatory process. They do not predispose to rampant superadded infection and it is only their abuse that leads to fungal overgrowth within the EAM. Antibiotic-containing drops should be avoided as these may cause further hypersensitivity of the EAM skin.

In severe cases with pain and marked occlusion of the canal, a deep intra-muscular 40-mg injection of Depo-Medrone (methylprednisolone acetate 40 mg/ml) is often helpful in reducing the pain and swelling. Systemic antibiotics should only be prescribed if there is surrounding cellulitis and lymphadenitis. Analgesia obviously should not be forgotten. Toilet should be performed as often as possible until the condition shows signs of abating. However, it is wise to continue the use of ear drops for a minimum period of 2 weeks.

Predisposing factors, when known, should be eliminated and avoided. Patients should be advised against the use of cotton buds and they should avoid getting water in their ears. They should not have their ears syringed (see section on Wax) and if they are avid swimmers, they should wear good-fitting ear plugs and a bathing cap if necessary.

Patients with otitis externa should be warned that the condition is difficult to treat, is often resistant to treatment and that recurrence is common. They should however be assured of the doctor's presence and willingness to help at these times.

Furuncle of the EAM

This is due to a staphylococcal infection of hair follicles in the EAM. The patient will complain of severe pain and impaired hearing if the canal is occluded by the swelling.

Examination reveals tenderness on traction of the pinna. A tender, red swelling may be seen in the external canal but often the canal is oedematous and occluded. There is usually associated peri-auricular lymphadenopathy.

Treatment involves the use of anti-staphylococcal antibiotics (flucloxacillin or erythromycin in penicillin-sensitive patients) and these almost always control this condition. Glycerine and ichthammol applied on a "ribbon gauze" wick is often soothing but there is no need for the liberal use of ear drops. Incision and drainage is hardly ever required. Once again, appropriate analgesia should not be forgotten as this is a very painful condition.

Perichondritis of the Pinna

This is an infective condition of the cartilage of the pinna. It may occur in isolation or as a continuum of otitis externa. It may also follow haematoma auris (see section on The Injured Ear) and frostbite and it occasionally follows surgery involving the cartilage of the pinna. Diabetes should be excluded.

Examination reveals a tender, hot, red pinna with surrounding cellulitis and lymphadenitis. Treatment involves the administration of parenteral antibiotics, incision and drainage where indicated and analgesia. Deformity of the pinna may be the end result of this condition. A small number of patients suffer a relapsing perichondritis of the pinna, the aetiology of which is unknown.

Herpes Infections

Herpes simplex may occur in the external ear and pinna and is particularly painful at these sites.

Bullous myringitis is an uncommon but painful condition which may occur in association with influenza. Haemorrhagic bullae are seen on the tympanic membrane and a conductive hearing loss often accompanies this disorder due to a concomitant middle-ear effusion.

Treatment involves the administration of antibiotics if bacterial superinfection is present or suspected. If these conditions are seen early in their course, both topical and systemic acyclovir (see Chap. 8) may be useful.

The Ramsay-Hunt syndrome (herpes zoster oticus) is a condition comprising severe pain of the pinna and external canal, vesicle formation at these sites, sensorineural hearing loss, vertigo and an ipsilateral facial nerve palsy (lower motor neurone). These patients should be referred for specialist ENT assessment once the diagnosis has been made.

Necrotising Otitis Externa (synonym: Malignant Otitis Externa)

This is a severe form of otitis externa that occurs in diabetic or immuno-suppressed patients. It is due to *Pseudomonas* infection which produces an underlying osteitis as well. Pain is usually severe and cranial nerve palsies may be associated presenting features. This condition requires urgent specialist referral as a significant number of these patients die.

Tumours of the EAM and Pinna

Benign tumours occurring in this area are the same as those found in the skin elsewhere. The tumours of greatest concern, however, are the basal cell carcinoma, which is locally destructive, and the squamous cell carcinoma, whose prognosis is particularly poor in this area.

Tumours of the EAM are on the whole uncommon. Malignant tumours are usually painful and there is almost always bony invasion present at the time of diagnosis. All such tumours should be referred for specialist assessment and treatment.

Diseases of the Middle Ear and Mastoid

Acute Otitis Media

This is an acute infective process of the middle ear which occurs most commonly in childhood. It often follows, or is part of, a viral upper respiratory tract infection. It is important to remember that the middle ear (via the Eustachian tube) is a continuation of the upper respiratory tract. While acute otitis media is usually viral in origin it may then become secondarily infected by bacteria normally resident in the upper respiratory tract. The commonest bacteria involved are streptococci, pneumococci and *H.influenzae*.

Although the patient is usually a child, this disease does rarely occur in adults. The presenting features include pyrexia, pain and irritability. If perforation of the tympanic membrane occurs, there is relief of the pain and consequent discharge of purulent middle-ear fluid. Older children and adults may complain of impaired hearing but this is obviously not a presenting feature in infants and toddlers.

Examination reveals a fretful child with a pyrexial illness. There may be erythema of the oropharynx or frank infection of either the tonsils, the pharynx or the nose (rhinitis). The pinna is not tender to traction and there is no peri-auricular lymphadenopathy. The external canal appears normal but the tympanic membrane is red and may bulge due to fluid accumulation in the middle ear. The light reflex is usually absent but the significance of the light reflex is often overemphasised. There is seldom a need to test for mobility of the drum as the diagnosis is usually clear. Insufflation of the drum would indeed be unnecessarily painful in this condition.

Management. Appropriate antibiotics in therapeutic doses against the most likely organisms (see above) should be given. However, there is considerable controversy regarding the duration of antibiotic administration and there has recently been a vogue for a "short, sharp" course of treatment. A 1-week course of treatment is probably a desirable minimum as inadequate treatment only leads to recurrence. Topical nasal decongestants are a valuable adjunct as they decongest the nasal airway and Eustachian tube. Systemic decongestants usually have side-effects and antihistamine preparations may complicate matters by increasing the viscosity of the middle-ear fluid. Analgesia and antipyretics should not be forgotten and symptoms should settle down within 48 hours of commencing treatment.

Feverish young children should be sponged down and continental quilts should be avoided as they are too effective in preventing heat loss from the pyrexial child.

Failure of resolution, perforations that do not heal within 4 weeks or other complications necessitate specialist referral.

Acute Mastoiditis

The mastoid is in continuity with the middle ear and is therefore always involved in acute otitis media. However, frank mastoiditis is fortunately an uncommon complication of this disease process. This is due to improved socio-economic conditions, early recognition and the prompt treatment of acute otitis media. If any of these factors are missing, as may occur in underprivileged communities, the incidence of acute mastoiditis rises.

The patient is again usually a child but adults may also be affected. There is pyrexia, malaise and irritability. There is tenderness over the mastoid antrum (Fig. 2.2) and extension of the suppurative process involves the mastoid cortex and periosteum. Pus may accumulate in the subperiosteal plane or the periosteum may be breached. The resultant post-auricular swelling pushes the pinna outwards and forwards. The tympanic membrane shows signs of the underlying inflammation, being either dull or red, and its mobility is reduced by the presence of fluid in the middle ear. However, the drum may be difficult to visualise in the very young patient or it may be obscured by wax.

Referral to an ENT department should be immediate as admission to hospital is mandatory for the appropriate treatment to be carried out.

The Discharging Ear

Discharge from the ear may be mucoid, mucopurulent, purulent or blood-stained. An appropriate history should be taken paying special attention to

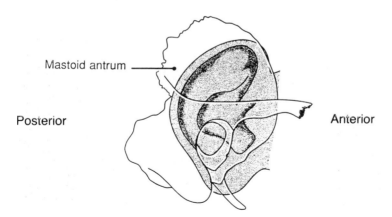

Mastoid antrum

Posterior

Anterior

Fig. 2.2. Surface marking of the mastoid antrum.

pain, previous surgery, swimming, cotton bud abuse and injury. It is then important to establish whether the discharge arises from the middle ear, external ear or rarely both. The presence of mucus in the discharge usually indicates the presence of a tympanic membrane perforation. Discharge of wax from the external canal may be confusing, especially in the pyrexial child. The high temperature may melt the wax causing it to appear as an "infected" discharge. The association of pyrexia and such a discharge from the ear may lead to a mistaken diagnosis of acute otitis media.

If the discharge is obscuring the view of the external canal and tympanic membrane, dry mopping of the ear should be performed. This is best done using a Jobson–Horne probe with some cotton wool lightly "fluffed" around the serrated end (Fig. 2.3). The loose end of the cotton wool is then used for mopping thus avoiding injury to the canal or drum with the probe itself. If however there is a history of trauma with associated bloody otorrhoea, any interference should be avoided for fear of converting an uninfected traumatic perforation into an infected one (see section on The Injured Ear).

Otitis Externa

See section on The Painful Ear.

Chronic Suppurative Otitis Media

This is a condition in which there is chronic suppuration of the middle-ear cleft (i.e. the middle ear and mastoid) associated with a perforation of the tympanic membrane. There has traditionally been a division of this disorder into tubo-tympanic disease and attico-antral disease (Table 2.1). In the past, tubo-tympanic disease has been labelled "safe" ear disease and not life-threatening, whereas attico-antral disease has been labelled "unsafe" and life-threatening.

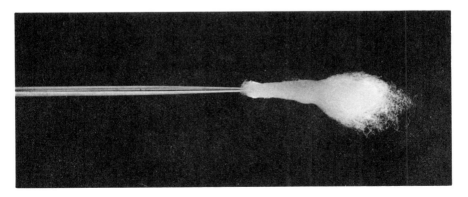

Fig. 2.3. Jobson–Horne probe with cotton wool. Used for dry mopping the EAM.

Table 2.1. Chronic suppurative otitis media

	Tubo-tympanic disease	Attico-antral disease
Perforation	Central	Marginal/posterior
Discharge	Profuse, mucopurulent	Scanty Foul smelling
Hearing loss	<35 db	>35 db
Cholesteatoma	Rare	Common

Practitioners should be aware that this is not absolutely true, as tubo-tympanic disease may also be unsafe and may also lead to intracranial complications. It is important to realise too that variations occur in both of the above conditions and none of the features listed in Table 2.1 is absolute or necessarily restricted to either variety of suppurative middle-ear disease.

The aim of the General Practitioner should be to make a diagnosis if possible, initiate treatment and refer these patients for specialist assessment. If it is impossible to make the diagnosis due to inability to visualise the tympanic membrane, the patient should be referred to an ENT surgeon for further management.

The ENT surgeon's management of patients with chronic suppurative otitis media involves cleaning out the ear with the aid of the operating microscope and suction apparatus, drying up the discharge and then attempting to prevent further episodes of infection. Cleaning the ear this way in the ENT department enables the ENT surgeon to make a definitive diagnosis. The state of the tympanic membrane and the middle ear can then be documented and the appropriate treatment commenced. A variety of ear drops can be used for this purpose and no single preparation has been shown to be superior to any other. It would appear though that the steroid component of the drops is the most active ingredient in achieving a dry ear. Bacterial swabs of the discharge are of little if any value as commensals and contaminants are usually cultured and the results of such investigations do not influence the management of the patient. Systemic antibiotics are unnecessary unless there is associated systemic illness (hardly ever) or intracranial complications.

Thus with aural toilet and topical treatment, a dry ear can be achieved in the majority of patients. The patient should also be advised against getting water in the ear as this often provokes infection or exacerbates infection that is already present.

The ENT surgeon must decide whether surgery is indicated or not. There is much controversy in this area but an outline of advised practice is presented.

In general a perforated tympanic membrane should be repaired. This operation is known as tympanoplasty. The aims of the operation are:

1. to repair the tympanic membrane;
2. to protect the middle ear; and ·
3. to restore the middle-ear conducting mechanism.

The majority of patients with perforated ear drums can and should be offered a repair of the drum although an 80 year old with ischaemic heart disease who has had a dry central perforation all his life would obviously not be a candidate for a tympanoplasty.

An important complication of chronic middle-ear disease is the development of cholesteatoma. This is an "epidermoid" cyst formed as a result of negative pressure occurring within the middle ear. This is usually due to Eustachian tube dysfunction, but localised areas of poor ventilation within the middle ear may be causative. A retraction "pocket" is then formed in the tympanic membrane and squamous epithelium accumulates within this pocket. This accumulation of squamous epithelium in conjunction with continued negative pressure enlarges the retraction pocket and by its medial expansion may cause erosion of the middle-ear components. This locally aggressive behaviour of cholesteatoma can further erode medially into the inner ear and through the thin plate of bone (tegmen) separating the middle ear from the cranial cavity. If this process is accompanied by infection, the disease behaves in a particularly aggressive fashion. Thus it can be seen how chronic suppurative otitis media can destroy the middle ear, the inner ear and lead to intracranial complications such as meningitis and intracranial abscesses. Hearing loss associated with this disease is due to tympanic membrane perforation, ossicular damage or inner-ear erosion. Cholesteatoma may also compress the facial nerve in its passage through the middle ear resulting in a facial nerve palsy. It is important to realise that cholesteatoma formation may be an insidious process and it may only present when intracranial complications have occurred.

The presence of cholesteatoma makes surgery mandatory and a variety of operations can be performed for this disease process (see Glossary).

Granular Myringitis

This is a condition in which there is inflammation of the tympanic membrane associated with small granulations on the drum itself. The cause of this condition is not known but it may be a variant of otitis externa. The granulations tend to produce a mucoid substance and this is the only condition of the external ear in which mucus is present in the absence of a tympanic membrane perforation.

The patient usually complains of pain although this is not as severe as in true otitis externa. There is discharge from the ear and a hearing loss is present, usually due to the fluid in the EAM.

Examination reveals a mucoid discharge in the external canal but the walls of the canal are not inflamed and the pinna is not tender to traction (see also section on Otitis Externa). There may be an underlying middle-ear effusion but this is difficult to diagnose in the presence of active disease of the tympanic membrane itself. A conductive hearing loss may be detected using a tuning fork.

Treatment involves aural toilet and the application of topical preparations (see Chap. 8). The condition is often resistant to treatment and may require several courses of topical applications. Spirit drops (90% ethyl alcohol) are often useful for drying out the ear and cautery of the granulations is sometimes effective in resistant cases.

The Diminished Hearing Ear

Impaired hearing may be due to a defective conducting mechanism, sensorineural problems or a combination of the two.

Conductive hearing loss is due to a defect in the conducting mechanism which carries sound waves to the inner ear. This may be due to absence or deformity of the pinna, obstruction of the EAM, disease of the tympanic membrane or ossicular problems. Ossicular problems may result from bone erosion (e.g. by cholesteatoma) with resultant ossicular discontinuity, from traumatic dislocation of the ossicles or from fixation of the ossicular chain.

Sensorineural hearing loss is due to impaired function of the cochlea and/or its neural connections.

Conductive Hearing Loss

Congenital Abnormalities

Congenital abnormalities of the pinna, EAM and middle ear are uncommon and should be referred to an ENT surgeon for further assessment.

Secretory Otitis Media ("Glue Ear")

This is a common condition occurring in young children. The higher incidence of upper respiratory tract infections in children leads to Eustachian tube dysfunction. This in turn produces a state of negative pressure within the middle ear which leads to the transudation of fluid from the lining cells of the middle-ear cleft. The fluid thus formed in the middle ear is of varying viscosity but it is often thick and gelatinous, hence the term "glue ear". This condition is by far the commonest cause of hearing loss in children.

There appears to be a bimodal distribution of the age incidence of children with "glue ears", the two peaks occurring at the time of teething and when children commence schooling.

These children arrive at the doctor with a variety of presenting problems. Delayed speech development may occur in younger children and infants with secretory otitis media may simply be "irritable". Some children may be referred to the doctor because they have failed the health visitor's screening tests for hearing loss. The parents may have noticed a hearing impairment and the teacher may report diminished hearing, behaviour problems or that scholastic performance has declined as a result of the hearing loss.

The majority of cases of "glue ear" (80%) will resolve spontaneously within 3 months. There is no proof that antibiotics, mucolytics or decongestants hasten or in any way influence this resolution rate. Antihistamines should be avoided (see Chap. 8). The remaining children in whom the condition does not resolve may require the insertion of ventilation tubes (grommets). A grommet is purely a ventilation tube and not a drainage tube. It is inserted into an incision in the tympanic membrane (Fig. 2.4) and serves to ventilate the middle-ear cleft. Grommets are eventually extruded by the ear itself. This may occur any time after their insertion but most grommets are extruded by 2 years. A small number of children (approximately 2%) have persistent otorrhoea through the grommet but this is easily dried up with a topical preparation such as Sofradex (see Chap. 8). Some children will also develop varying degrees of tympanosclerosis (white chalk-like plaques) in the tympanic membrane but this does not appear to be of any significance.

Parents will usually enquire about swimming and grommets. There is considerable variation of opinion in this regard. At opposite ends of the spectrum, some ENT surgeons will forbid a single drop of water to enter the ear whilst others will simply suggest that excessive water should not enter the EAM. Thus parents should be warned that water may be harmful and that it should not be liberally splashed around the ear canal, e.g. when washing the child's hair. As regards swimming, if the child wears good ear plugs with a bathing cap and does not indulge in diving, there should not be any problems. If otorrhoea does occur despite these precautions then swimming should cease.

Perforations of the Tympanic Membrane

Perforations of the tympanic membrane are a common cause of conductive hearing loss. They are discussed under The Discharging Ear and The Injured Ear.

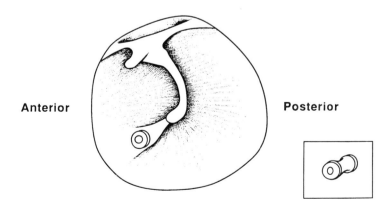

Anterior　　　　　　　　　　　　　　　　**Posterior**

Fig. 2.4. Grommet in situ. *Inset* Grommet.

Ossicular Discontinuity

Skull trauma or a blow to the side of the head may cause dislocation and discontinuity of the ossicular chain. There may or may not be an associated perforation of the tympanic membrane. If a conductive hearing loss persists for longer than 3 months after such an injury, surgical repair of the ossicular chain (ossiculoplasty) can be performed.

Wax

It is a normal phenomenon for the ceruminous glands of the external ear to produce wax, which normally clears spontaneously from the EAM. However, many patients are obsessed with the desire to have it removed. Wax is not nearly as common a cause of hearing loss as is generally believed by patients. If the external canal is plugged with excessive wax, a conductive hearing loss may indeed result but most patients with abundant external canal wax have normal hearing.

If there is a need to remove wax, this may be done by syringing provided there is no history of tympanic membrane perforation, previous ear surgery or otitis externa. In these circumstances syringing may cause a flare-up of any disease process present and it may convert a dry ear into a discharging ear.

If there is doubt or difficulty in removing wax, suction clearance with the aid of the operating microscope can be performed in the local ENT department. Hard wax may be softened by instilling olive oil or sodium bicarbonate drops into the ear for a few days prior to attempted removal. Cotton buds and other implements such as hair grips should be forbidden as they cause injury and push the wax even deeper into the external canal.

Foreign Bodies

These should be gently removed by syringing or using appropriate instrumentation. If any difficulty is encountered, the patient should be referred for specialist management. This policy will prevent unnecessary injury to the external canal and tympanic membrane.

Otosclerosis

This condition is a localised disease of the ear in which new "spongy" bone is deposited around the stapes footplate. It may be unilateral or bilateral. The resultant immobility of the stapes impedes sound transmission to the inner ear producing a conductive hearing loss.

The onset of the hearing loss is gradually noticed in the third decade and approximately 50% of these patients have a family history of the disorder. Examination shows the tympanic membrane to be normal but tuning fork tests and formal audiometry reveal the presence of a conductive hearing loss. Patients with otosclerosis may be offered a hearing aid or a surgical procedure known as stapedectomy (see Glossary).

Exostoses

These bony outgrowths in the external canal are covered by skin and may grow large enough to occlude the canal. Debris may accumulate medial to these structures leading to otitis externa or obstruction. Their very size may cause a conductive hearing loss. Surgical removal is only indicated if such complications occur. They are most common in swimmers and surfers.

Sensorineural Hearing Loss

This type of hearing loss may be due to cochlear disorders, auditory nerve problems or a combination of the two.

Presbycusis

This is the hearing loss associated with increasing age. The age of onset varies from one individual to another and is probably influenced by genetic and environmental factors. It is the commonest type of hearing loss affecting man.

Examination reveals normal tympanic membranes but hearing tests reveal a sensorineural hearing loss, especially affecting the higher frequencies. Other otological problems must be excluded before the rehabilitation of these patients is commenced. This is rehabilitation in its broadest sense to prevent these patients from becoming socially isolated. They should be assessed for their suitability to wear a hearing aid and although hearing aids are not a panacea for this condition, many of these patients can be helped significantly with such a device. This is largely due to improved technology in the production of hearing aids. Hearing aids are essentially of two types:

1. Body-worn hearing aids: air conduction aids or bone conduction aids.
2. Ear-level aids: ear-level aids are either worn post-aurally or may be inserted in the ear itself.

Body-worn aids are the more "old-fashioned" type of hearing aids which are attached by a clip to an item of the patient's clothing. The receiver is fitted to the ear-mould and is attached by a lead to the hearing aid. They are still used in the patient with a particularly severe hearing loss as they allow considerable amplification without "feedback" problems as occurs in "ear-level" aids when amplification is excessive. They are more conspicuous and are also susceptible to interference due to friction with the patient's clothing. They are however easier to use when the patient has problems of dexterity, e.g. rheumatoid arthritis affecting the hands.

Ear-level aids are air-conduction hearing aids, whereby sound is transmitted to the cochlea via the external ear canal. Air-conduction aids are used when there is no otorrhoea and these devices are worn either post-aurally as prescribed in the NHS or they may be worn completely within the ear canal. The latter type are not available on the NHS as they are considerably more expensive. Their main advantage is cosmetic in that the device is less visible than the post-aural aid although the post-aural aid can be hidden by the patient's hair.

A bone-conduction hearing aid is worn either as a headband or on the arms of a pair of spectacles. They are useful in the presence of a discharging ear because a device occluding the ear canal aggravates the otorrhoea. Bone-conduction aids require firm apposition to the skull for effective transmission of sound and this tight fitting may be somewhat uncomfortable for the patient.

A small number of patients in whom there is good cochlea function, but in whom an ear-level aid would be unsuitable, may benefit from an implantable hearing aid. This includes patients who have absent or deformed pinnae, various degrees of external canal atresia or chronically discharging ears. However, the device, which is embedded in the skull bone via a post-aural incision, is expensive and is not as yet available on the NHS. It must also be emphasised that only a small number of patients are suitable to have such a device implanted.

A small number of patients with a profound bilateral sensorineural hearing loss may benefit from the insertion of a cochlear implant. This device must still be considered to be experimental and is only available in a few selected centres.

Supply of a hearing aid depends on the needs of the patient, i.e. their home circumstances, occupation etc. and these factors should therefore always be taken into consideration.

Several environmental aids are available which provide amplification to the doorbell, telephone and television. Lip reading may also be extremely valuable and most ENT departments either provide lip-reading classes or will advise patients on where this skill can be learned (see Appendix). In addition, some ENT departments have the services of a hearing therapist who is able to provide auditory training for patients with hearing problems.

Noise-Induced Hearing Loss

This condition arises from prolonged exposure to excessive noise. The hearing loss usually occurs in patients who have been exposed to excessive noise levels, for example working in noisy factories, operating noisy machinery, firing weapons etc.

Prevention of exposure to these noise levels is the prime aim and involves decreasing the ambient noise where possible or the use of ear defenders if ambient noise remains excessive. Once a hearing loss of this kind has occurred, it is not reversible. Patients who have a suspected noise-induced hearing loss may be eligible for compensation and would require assessment by an ENT surgeon and an audiologist for such a case to be considered.

Drug-Induced Hearing Loss

Systemic administration of aminoglycoside antibiotics, some diuretics and cytotoxic drugs may lead to sensorineural hearing loss. Ototoxicity associated with the former two groups of drugs is usually associated with abnormally elevated blood levels of the drug. Correspondingly high levels of the drugs are then found in the inner-ear fluids as well. This may arise from over-zealous prescribing but is more commonly due to impaired renal function which leads to reduced excretion of the drugs. It is therefore imperative that if these drugs are being administered, especially in the presence of impaired renal function, blood levels of the drugs are measured at the appropriate times in relation to administration. Cytotoxic drugs appear to have a more direct effect on the cochlea and the damage produced is not always dose-related. Toxic levels of salicylates may produce a hearing loss but this is usually transient and reversible.

Topical antibiotics used in chronic suppurative otitis media have often been thought or said to be toxic to the inner ear. However, there is no evidence of this being so in humans.

Congenital Hearing Loss

Such a hearing loss may be due to genetic factors or due to maternal illness in pregnancy. Rubella is the best known of the latter group. The incidence of congenital hearing loss due to rubella has decreased in developed countries due to increased awareness of the condition and the active immunisation of adolescent females against the rubella virus. It is important for any woman planning a pregnancy to undergo a serological test for rubella antibodies. If she has no antibodies, she may well be advised to have a rubella vaccination at least 3 months before conception takes place. Other viral illnesses or syphilis may also be responsible for a congenital hearing loss. Although the hearing defect is permanent, early recognition is crucial to maximally utilise any hearing present and to ensure that the necessary supportive and educational measures are commenced at an early age thereby ensuring the child's integration into society (see Appendix).

Sudden Sensorineural Hearing Loss

Any sudden loss of hearing (usually a substantial or total unilateral loss) should be referred for special assessment. In most cases the cause is unknown although it may be of viral origin. A small number of cases are due to conditions which may be amenable to treatment. These include hypercoagulable haematological disorders, spontaneous rupture of the round window and, rarely, acoustic neuroma. To permit the early detection of a treatable cause and to then commence treatment, it is imperative that these patients are referred as a matter of urgency.

Acoustic Neuroma

This is a rare benign tumour of the VIIIth cranial nerve. It may present with a variety of symptoms which include hearing loss, tinnitus and, rarely, vertigo. Symptoms of raised intracranial pressure are a late presentation of a large tumour. Acoustic neuroma is an uncommon cause of these symptoms but ENT surgeons are always vigilant for its presentation. If diagnosed early, it can usually be removed relatively safely by ENT surgeons or neurosurgeons. If it is

25

diagnosed when it has attained a larger size, the risks associated with the requisite neurosurgical procedure are far greater. Although benign in a histopathological sense, its site of occurrence (along the path of the vestibulocochlear nerve) makes it potentially lethal, especially if diagnosed late.

Syphilis

Tertiary or neurosyphilis causes a sensorineural hearing loss. All patients with an unexplained sensorineural hearing loss should have serological tests for syphilis. Both the treatment for otoneurosyphilis and the success rates for such treatment are controversial. The treatment should be undertaken by the specialist and usually involves the administration of anti-syphilitic antibiotics and steroids.

Other Infections

Measles, mumps, meningitis and influenza may all produce a sensorineural hearing loss due to cochlear or VIIIth nerve damage. Active immunisation against measles and mumps will reduce the incidence of hearing loss produced by these diseases. Any patient who has had meningitis should undergo audiometric testing after recovery from their illness. In this way any hearing loss suffered as a result of the illness can be detected and the appropriate rehabilitation measures commenced.

Non-organic Hearing Loss

A small number of people will feign a hearing loss. They usually complain of a unilateral hearing loss which is often total. This may be hysterical in nature or may arise out of a desire for financial compensation. The latter group may be claiming compensation either for noise-induced hearing loss or following trauma to the skull or ear.

Some adolescents with emotional problems may also present with an apparent hearing loss.

Malingering can usually be uncovered by a skilled audiologist or otologist.

The Injured Ear

Injury to the ear may involve the pinna, the external canal, the tympanic membrane, the ossicles or the inner ear. These structures may be injured singly or in combination.

The Pinna

Injuries to the pinna may be blunt or sharp. Blunt injury is the type commonly seen in rugby forwards and boxers and results in the accumulation of blood deep to the perichondrium of the pinna. As the blood supply of the underlying cartilage is largely derived from this covering layer, their resultant separation leads to eventual necrosis of the cartilage. The acute condition is known as haematoma auris and the resulting deformity is commonly referred to as a "cauliflower ear". Haematoma auris requires immediate drainage and a firm pressure dressing to prevent the re-accumulation of the haematoma and to re-appose the perichondrium to the cartilage.

Lacerations of the pinna should be sutured early obtaining as good a cosmetic result as possible. Any exposed cartilage should be covered with skin.

The External Canal

Injuries to the external canal are most commonly self-inflicted resulting from the patient's attempts to clean or scratch his own ear. These minor abrasions or lacerations usually heal spontaneously.

The Tympanic Membrane

Injury to the ear drum may result from a blow to the ear, from over-zealous attempts to clean the ear (by patient or doctor) or from a nearby blast. Over 80% of traumatic perforations of the tympanic membrane will heal spontaneously provided the ear is kept clean and dry. When such patients are seen in the acute phase, no attempt should be made to remove blood clot from the external meatus. If there is any doubt about the extent or severity of the injury, a specialist opinion should be sought as a matter of urgency. Syringing such ears is strongly contraindicated and ear drops are generally unnecessary unless infection supervenes. If the perforation has not healed within 3 months, the patient should be offered a repair of the tympanic membrane (tympanoplasty).

The Ossicles

The same agents that cause tympanic membrane injury may be responsible for causing ossicular discontinuity. The same principles of management pertain as in injury to the tympanic membrane. Occasionally ossicular discontinuity may occur following injury without damage to the drum itself. This may be visible on otoscopy or a conductive hearing loss may ensue following the injury. Such ossicular damage can be surgically repaired (see also section on Conductive Hearing Loss – Ossicular Discontinuity).

The Inner Ear

Severe head injury, blast trauma or excessive noise may all injure the inner ear. Damage to the inner ear in these conditions usually results in a permanent sensorineural hearing loss. Those in whom the sensorineural hearing loss recovers (the minority) can be retrospectively diagnosed as having suffered "labyrinthine concussion".

Patients with severe head injuries may also have injuries to all or some of the above-mentioned structures. Such patients obviously require complete assessment of all their injuries and always require hospitalisation.

The Noisy Ear

Noises in the ear (tinnitus) may be heard by the patient alone – subjective tinnitus, or they may be audible to the examining doctor as well – objective tinnitus. The latter may be heard by placing the examining ear close to where the patient describes the origin of the sound or by using a stethoscope at the same site. The commonly described noises of tinnitus include ringing, buzzing or pulsating sounds. Complex noises such as voices, orchestras etc. usually indicate some psychological disturbance rather than an otological disorder.

Tinnitus is often a very bothersome symptom for the patient and may itself lead to severe psychological disturbance. It is almost always associated with some degree of sensorineural hearing loss. Patients with tinnitus require a great deal of emotional support and the exclusion of any disease process is often of great comfort to them. The majority of these patients have no known cause for their symptoms but a small minority have a disease process in the ear or surrounding structures producing tinnitus. Many patients are concerned that they may have a brain tumour and indeed tumours of the internal auditory meatus and cerebello-pontine angle must be excluded. These patients therefore require specialist referral to exclude a treatable disorder and to introduce them to the support services (see Appendix) available for tinnitus sufferers. Tinnitus can often be masked by the provision of background noise. This can be achieved by the radio, personal stereo sets, tinnitus maskers or merely a hearing aid.

Objective tinnitus may be due to arteriovenous malformations in the vicinity of the ear, glomus jugulare tumours or rarely when a flying insect has lodged itself in the external canal. The first two require specialist management whilst an insect can be removed with forceps or by syringing.

By far the majority of patients with tinnitus have subjective tinnitus with no demonstrable cause for their distressing symptoms.

The Cosmetic Ear

The commonest condition requiring cosmetic surgery is that known as "bat ears". Children with such ears that are placed almost at 90° to the side of the head may suffer embarrassment and be subjected to constant mockery at school. This condition is treatable by an operation known as pinnaplasty which is performed by ENT surgeons and plastic surgeons alike.

Varying degrees of agenesis or atresia of the external ear should be referred for specialist assessment as they may be associated with middle- and inner-ear abnormalities as well.

3 The Dizzy Patient

Dizziness is a common complaint and one which causes a great deal of alarm for the patient. Although dizziness means different things to different people, the actual symptom whereby the patient is unable to control his equilibrium is very disturbing to him.

When a patient complains of dizziness, the doctor's prime objective is to establish what the patient means. If the patient is describing symptoms of "feeling faint" or "about to black out" this is not vertigo. Postural hypotension is unlikely to be the cause of vestibular problems. Thus the doctor needs to find out whether the dizzy patient is in fact suffering from vertigo. It is the symptom of vertigo that concerns the ENT surgeon and this may be defined as an hallucination or illusion of movement, with or without rotatory symptoms. Once the symptom of true vertigo has been elicited, an attempt is then made to assess whether the symptom arises from peripheral receptors such as the vestibule of the inner ear, or whether it is central (i.e. central nervous system) in origin.

Vertigo arises as a result of abnormal stimulation of the sense organs responsible for maintaining the body's equilibrium. The body's equilibrium is maintained by the vestibule of the inner ear, various nerve pathways in the brain and spinal cord, the eyes, joints, muscles and tendons. All these organs respond to the body's position in space and by complex interaction keep us in a state of equilibrium.

In the majority of patients, the diagnosis can be made by taking the history. This requires patience and the avoidance of leading questions.

The following questions are relevant: "Can you describe exactly what you feel when you feel dizzy?"; "How long does the dizziness last?"; "How often does it occur?"; "Does anything bring the dizziness on?"; "Does anything relieve the dizziness?" It is also important to know whether there is associated nausea or vomiting. The presence of these features not only points to the severity of the symptoms, but is more commonly associated with true vertigo than with other vague symptoms described as dizziness. Other questions of relevance refer to cardiovascular disease, otological problems in the past, head injury and any medication currently being taken.

The history is thus an attempt to establish whether there is true vertigo or not and, if there is, to establish whether it is of vestibular or central origin.

The examination is seldom contributory and will either fail to demonstrate any physical signs or will confirm the diagnosis assumed from the patient's history.

Examination should include measurement of the patient's blood pressure in the erect and supine positions and an evaluation of the cardiovascular system. A full ENT examination should be performed paying special attention to the ears. A neurological examination should then be carried out to look for evidence of a central or vestibular disturbance. The cranial nerves should be examined in turn, the presence or absence of nystagmus noted, cerebellar signs should be sought and the posterior columns' function observed. The hearing should also be tested with tuning forks.

Special investigations should be left to the specialist clinic, whether this be the neurology or the ENT clinic. These tests will include a full blood count and sedimentation rate (or blood viscosity), audiometry, electronystagmography and calorics where indicated and appropriate radiological investigations.

Before describing various causative conditions, it is important to recall that the VIIIth cranial nerve has both vestibular and cochlear elements and that the inner ear is similarly divided. Thus disorders of balance arising in these areas may affect the vestibular section alone or may involve the cochlea as well.

Vestibular Neuronitis

This is a disorder in which only the vestibular portion of the inner ear (not the cochlea), specifically the vestibular nerve, is thought to be involved. There is often a preceding history of an upper respiratory tract infection and for this reason the condition is thought to be viral in origin. The patient experiences vertigo, nausea and vomiting but his hearing is unaffected. The diagnosis is one of exclusion. Treatment involves reassurance and the use of vestibular sedatives such as prochlorperazine or cinnarizine (see Chap. 8). Prochlorperazine may often have to be given parenterally in the early stages (first 24–48 hours) as the vomiting and vertigo can be particularly severe. Recovery is the normal end result but this may take several months.

Positional Vertigo (synonyms: Benign Paroxysmal Positional Vertigo; Cupulolithiasis)

In this disorder the patient has paroxysmal attacks of vertigo, which are precipitated by changes in the position of the head. The attacks are usually short lived. They may wake the patient from sleep as a result of turning in bed and rapidly turning the head to look at oncoming traffic may precipitate an attack. Some patients have a history of head injury but this is so in less than 50% of patients with this disorder.

There is no associated hearing loss and while nausea and vomiting may occur, they are not prominent features as the symptoms are short lived.

Positional nystagmus is diagnostic but once again the diagnosis is usually made from the history. The nystagmus is also fatiguable.

Patients should be reassured that this is a benign disorder which is usually self-limiting although recurrent. Patients often learn to avoid manoeuvres that precipitate attacks but vestibular sedatives may be necessary.

Labyrinthitis

Both the cochlear and the vestibular portions of the inner ear constitute the labyrinth. Inflammation of the labyrinth will therefore cause vertigo and hearing loss. A viral upper respiratory tract infection may be associated with labyrinthitis. The effects are usually temporary, lasting up to 6 weeks, but they may be permanent.

Chronic suppurative otitis media that spreads medially to involve the inner ear will usually result in a suppurative labyrinthitis. This is particularly so when cholesteatoma is present and usually necessitates surgical exploration and drainage. The end result in such patients is usually a non-hearing or "dead" ear.

Drugs

Several drugs may cause vertiginous symptoms. These include hypnotics, anti-convulsants, anti-parkinsonian drugs and the major tranquillisers.

Anti-hypertensive drugs may cause postural hypotension and syncope and thus feelings of faintness, but not true vertigo. The aminoglycoside antibiotics are ototoxic and have particular affinity for the vestibular end organs in the inner ear, especially in large doses. Therefore the administration of such drugs should be accompanied by accurate monitoring of serum drug levels.

Ménière's Disease

This disorder is made up of a triad of symptoms comprising tinnitus, vertigo and sensorineural hearing loss. It is not a common cause of vertigo and is probably over-diagnosed. The aetiology is unknown. The pathophysiology involves hydrops of the membranous labyrinth. Attacks are paroxysmal and the deafness and tinnitus are initially unilateral. However, the disease eventually becomes bilateral in over 50% of patients. The sensorineural hearing loss is

33

progressive and permanent. The vertiginous attacks are usually severe and are associated with nausea and vomiting.

Reassurance is essential for these patients and it is useful for them to see the same doctor whenever possible, and thus establish a rapport.

Drugs used include vasodilators such as nicotinic acid and betahistine, vestibular sedatives such a prochlorperazine and cinnarizine and diuretics such as the thiazides or carbonic anhydrase inhibitors (acetazolamide). Caffeine should be avoided and salt intake should be restricted.

Surgery is reserved for severe cases and the multitude of procedures used attests to the lack of agreement on the correct treatment.

Destructive procedures include labyrinthectomy or vestibular nerve section. Decompression procedures include endolymphatic sac decompression or shunting.

A diagnosis of Ménière's disease warrants referral to an ENT surgeon.

Acoustic Neuroma (see also Chap. 2)

The term "acoustic neuroma" is actually a misnomer as the tumour is a vestibulo-cochlear schwannoma that primarily involves the vestibular portion of the VIIIth cranial nerve. The involvement of this nerve may therefore give rise to vestibular symptoms.

It is important to put this into perspective and to appreciate that the "acoustic neuroma" is a rare tumour and subsequently a very rare cause of vertigo.

4 The Nose

Patients complain of a variety of nasal symptoms. However, the patient's complaints may bear little relation to the clinical findings, e.g. a patient complaining of a blocked nose may have an apparently patent airway whilst a patient with an apparently obstructed nasal airway may have no subjective symptoms of nasal obstruction.

The Blocked Nose

Nasal obstruction is a common complaint and may or may not be associated with nasal discharge (synonyms: "runny nose", rhinorrhoea). The history is very important as this often gives a clue as to whether this is a functional or purely mechanical obstruction. The age of the patient is relevant as nasal polyps are extremely rare in children whereas foreign bodies are uncommon in normal adults. The periodicity of the obstruction is important. Is it intermittent or constant? Is there a seasonal variation? Are there aggravating or relieving factors, e.g. temperature variations, anxiety, air-conditioning, foodstuffs? Is there associated rhinorrhoea? Is there a history of sneezing? Is there a history of trauma? Has there been topical decongestant abuse? Has there been any previous nasal surgery?

Vasomotor Rhinitis

Pure vasomotor rhinitis may be defined as a hypersensitivity of the nasal and paranasal mucosa to various stimuli. This hypersensitivity may be associated with predominance of either sympathetic or parasympathetic outflow leading to a "stuffy" nose in the former or a "runny" nose in the latter. It should be established whether the patient is not merely describing the changes that occur in the normal nasal cycle. There is a normal daily cyclical vasodilatation and vasoconstriction of the nasal mucosa which may cause a sensation of congestion in the vasodilator phase.

Thereafter patients should be treated with topical inhaled steroids in order to reduce the incidence of recurrence. It is uncertain how long this treatment should persist but 6 months is probably a minimum requirement.

There has been a recent vogue favouring the medical treatment of polyps with inhaled stereoids. However, the results are inconsistent and, at present, surgical removal is the treatment of choice.

Mechanical Obstruction

It is convenient to divide this group into the classical categories of congenital, traumatic, inflammatory, neoplastic and miscellaneous.

Congenital

Choanal Atresia. This is a rare condition of neonates in which an atretic plate of bone and/or mucosa obstructs the posterior nares of the nose. It may be unilateral or bilateral. In bilateral cases these infants present in the neonatal period with respiratory obstruction because neonates are obligatory nose-breathers. They require urgent referral to an ENT surgeon. Unilateral cases usually present in later life with unilateral rhinorrhoea and surgical correction can then be performed. Repair of choanal atresia may be performed trans-nasally or via a transpalatal approach.

Septal Deviation. This may present early in life or in adulthood. Treatment by surgical correction is only indicated if the deviation is causing symptomatic obstruction.

Traumatic

See section on The Injured Nose.

Inflammatory

See sections on Sinusitis and Nasal Polyps.

Neoplastic

Tumours of the nose and paranasal sinuses are rare and may present with nasal obstruction/discharge, epiphora (if the nasolacrimal duct is obstructed), facial pain or dental problems (if the upper jaw is involved) and hypoaesthesia of the cheek if the infraorbital nerve has been involved.

These patients should all be referred for specialist assessment and treatment. Treatment may involve radiotherapy, surgery and chemotherapy depending on the extent of the disease and its histological nature.

Miscellaneous

Rhinitis Medicamentosa. This condition results from the abuse of topical nasal decongestants. There is a drying out of the nasal mucosa with sensations of nasal obstruction and anosmia. Treatment involves immediate discontinuation of use of the offending agent. The patient should be advised that withdrawing the nose drops will produce further sensations of obstruction but that this will usually settle down spontaneously. Glucose and glycerine nose drops may be used in the interim to keep the nasal mucosa moist and free from further crust formation.

Adenoids. Enlarged adenoids (often together with enlarged tonsils) are a common cause of nasal obstruction in children. There may be a history of snoring, mouth-breathing, disturbed sleep pattern, difficult behaviour and daytime somnolence. A history of sleep apnoea may be volunteered by the parents but if not, such a history should be sought.

Sleep apnoea is characterised by episodes during sleep when breathing stops for short periods and then recommences. These children often snore excessively and the parents erroneously think that they are heavy or deep sleepers when in fact these periods of hypoxia actually disrupt their sleep pattern. This episodic hypoxia may lead to cardiac dysrhythmias, pulmonary hypertension or right-heart failure. Such children should be referred fairly urgently for assessment and adenoidectomy (with or without tonsillectomy) should be performed with relative urgency by the ENT team.

Snoring in adults is usually due to mechanical or functional obstruction of the upper airway (from the tip of the nose to the tracheal bifurcation) and can, in severe cases, lead to the same problems listed above (see section on Adenoids). In addition, excessive snoring may lead to marital stress and breakdown. Such cases also require ENT assessment. If no specific mechanical obstruction is found, an operation called uvulopalatopharyngoplasty can be performed. This involves the removal of redundant and lax tissues from the tonsillar pillars and soft palate.

The "Runny" Nose

Discharge from the nose may be watery, mucoid, mucopurulent, purulent or bloodstained. Watery rhinorrhoea is encountered in the early stages of the common cold, in allergic rhinitis and in the parasympathetic dominant variety of vasomotor rhinitis.

Vasomotor Rhinitis (see also section on The Blocked Nose)

This variant may be troublesome in that some patients actually have "water" dripping from their noses. This occurs largely in elderly patients. There has been some success with the use of ipratropium nasal spray (anti-cholinergic) but again the "drying-up" systemic agents such as antihistamines have the limitations mentioned above (see section on The Blocked Nose). Cautery of the inferior turbinates can be used to destroy receptor areas on the turbinates and may be successful in troublesome cases. However, the regenerative powers of the autonomic nervous system may render this relief only temporary.

Allergic Rhinitis

See section on The Blocked Nose.

Sinusitis

There is a lot of confusion about this condition and one is often greeted by patients who have "sinus", "sinusitis" or "chronic sinusitis". The entity needs to be clearly defined and appropriately managed. Sinusitis is an inflammatory (usually infective) condition of the paranasal sinuses which usually follows a viral infection of the upper respiratory tract. In the acute stage there is pyrexia, mucopurulent rhinorrhoea (anterior and/or posterior) and facial pain in the area of the involved sinus. Several other nasal and non-nasal (see Chap. 5) conditions are thus erroneously labelled as sinusitis.

It is worth remembering that all the paranasal sinuses except the frontal sinuses are present at birth. The frontal sinuses develop in childhood to reach a maximum size at puberty. However, failure of pneumatisation of one or both frontal sinuses may occur. This occurs much less commonly in the sphenoid and maxillary sinuses.

Management

Antibiotics should be prescribed against the commonest responsible pathogens (e.g. streptococci, *H. influenzae*) and also anaerobes if the infection is thought to be of dental origin. Topical decongestants (e.g. xylometazoline) are immensely valuable as they open the sinus ostium thereby facilitating natural drainage. Systemic decongestants add very little to the management of sinusitis and their side-effects probably make their added prescription unnecessary. Sinus X-rays in acute sinusitis are superfluous and are an unnecessary expense initially as they will not alter treatment. Treatment should probably continue for 10 days to 2 weeks.

Failure of treatment may be due to a resistant organism, the wrong antibiotic, or persistent obstruction of the natural ostium. If there is no response to treatment it is worth changing antibiotics. However, persistent obstruction of the sinus ostium may require surgical drainage. If symptoms are particularly severe at any stage, surgical drainage may be indicated. This would involve referral to an ENT surgeon who would perform the procedure (antrum wash-out) under either local or general anaesthesia. When treatment has failed, this would be an appropriate time to perform X-rays of the sinuses as this would help assess the response to therapy to date. Persistent and repeated obstruction of the sinus ostium may be due to anatomical problems within the nose such as a deviated septum. Correction of the deformity may also therefore be indicated but would normally be performed after the acute episode has been appropriately treated.

Foreign Body

This is usually associated with a foul-smelling, unilateral nasal discharge which may be blood-stained. Removal may be possible in the GP's surgery but any difficulty encountered in removal should prevent further action. The patient, usually a child, should then be referred to an ENT surgeon for assessment. With better facilities removal may be possible or a general anaesthetic may be required.

A bloody nasal discharge may be the presenting feature of a nasal tumour. Tumours of the nose and paranasal sinuses are rare but should nevertheless be considered in the presence of an unexplained bloody nasal discharge. (See also the section on The Blocked Nose – Mechanical Obstruction.)

The Injured Nose

Injuries to the nose cause cosmetic deformity and/or nasal obstruction. Fractures only require reduction if there is a cosmetic deformity which is unacceptable to the patient, if there is resultant nasal obstruction or if there is persistent epistaxis following the injury. The ideal time to reduce a nasal fracture is 7–10 days after the injury. Referral to the ENT surgeon should therefore occur before this time interval has elapsed. In the acute post-injury phase it is mandatory to examine the septum for a septal haematoma. This is easily done by elevating the tip of the nose or gently inserting a Thudicum speculum into the anterior nares. In the presence of such an injury the septum is markedly swollen, usually bilaterally, and the swelling usually fills both nostrils. Diagnosis of a septal haematoma requires an emergency referral (same day) for incision and drainage. Failure to do so may lead to the formation of septal abscess, destruction of the septum and consequent cosmetic deformity.

X-rays play very little part in the diagnosis or management of nasal fractures and are only used for medico-legal purposes.

The Bleeding Nose

The majority of nosebleeds arise from Little's area and stop with simple first-aid measures such as external pressure or the application of cold compresses of various sorts. Little's area is found at the anterior end of the septum just posterior to the mucocutaneous junction and can be examined by elevating the tip of the nose or with a Thudicum speculum.

How does the non-ENT surgeon manage a nosebleed that arises posteriorly or one that does not stop spontaneously?

The ideal solution is to identify the bleeding point and then cauterise it or tamponade it with the minimum amount of pressure necessary. Cautery may be performed by chemical means (silver nitrate or trichloracetic acid) or by electrocautery. The above measures require a good light source, suction, cautery facilities and appropriate packing materials, not to mention the required skills! If the bleeding point is visible, it should be cauterised. If it cannot be seen and the bleeding is continuing, the nose should be packed. Various packing materials may be used and these include BIPP (bismuth iodoform paraffin paste) and Merocel tampons among others. The majority of nosebleeds are unilateral and therefore require packing of the involved nostril only. In most cases when the bleeding appears to be bilateral, this is due to blood pouring around the posterior end of the septum into the other nostril. If packing still fails to control the bleeding the patient should be referred to an ENT department.

Excessive and indiscriminate cautery and packing of the nose will traumatise the entire nasal mucosa and prevent accurate identification of the true bleeding point. This is particularly important in patients with a generalised bleeding tendency.

The "I Can't Smell" Nose

Several patients complain of this symptom. Again the history is important and examination should exclude mechanical obstruction as a cause of anosmia. Treatment of conditions such as allergic rhinitis and nasal polyps will often restore the sense of smell. Permanent loss of smell may occur after "influenzal neuritis" involving the olfactory nerves. Basal skull fracture or intracranial lesions may also cause damage to the Ist cranial nerves but these are not common causes of anosmia. When no cause is found, it may be worthwhile to use inhaled steroids (e.g. beclomethasone or flunisolide) on an empirical basis as some patients report improvement with these measures.

The Cosmetic Nose

Rhinoplastic surgery is performed by both ENT surgeons and plastic surgeons. The deformity may involve the external skeleton of the nose and the septum.

Referral of patients requesting cosmetic surgery requires detailed discussion of the psychological factors involved. These include distorted body image, underlying feelings of inadequacy etc. It is important not to reject the patient and appear to dismiss his/her concern.

Other Conditions

Furunculosis

This is a staphylococcal infection of the nasal vestibule. Treatment involves the administration of systemic anti-staphylococcal antibiotics. Topical antibiotics or antiseptics have only a secondary role in this condition.

Rhinophyma

This condition occurs as a result of fibrosis and hyperplasia of the sebaceous glands on the dorsum of the nose. It usually arises as a consequence of acne rosacea and leads to marked swelling of the nose. Treatment may involve shaving off the excess tissue in severe cases and this may be done by a plastic surgeon or an ENT surgeon.

Wegener's Granulomatosis

This is a rare condition of unknown aetiology. The pathological process is that of a vasculitis with granuloma formation and the condition primarily affects the upper respiratory tract, the lungs and the kidneys. The presenting features in the nose therefore include nasal obstruction, bleeding and excessive crusting. The potential for destruction of the nasal cartilage is great and early biopsy of the offending lesion should be performed. Wegener's granulomatosis used to be almost uniformly fatal as patients developed renal failure as part of the disorder. However, treatment with steroids and immunosuppressive drugs such as cyclophosphamide and azathioprine have reversed this trend and most patients now survive. Plastic reconstructive procedures may be necessary to repair any resultant deformity of the nose, but this should wait until the disease process is in remission.

5 Facial Pain

Pain in the face not only arises from many different sites but may also be referred from distant sites (see Chap. 2, section on The Painful Ear). The history is all important and special note should be taken of the onset of the pain, its site, its periodicity and also of precipitating and relieving factors. Examination must then include inspection of the mouth and throat. The teeth should all be percussed to elicit tenderness lest the problem be of dental origin. The nose and ears should also be examined and the temporo-mandibular joints should be palpated. The neck should be palpated and finally the skin of the face should be tested for hypo- or hyperaesthesia. Particular attention should be paid to the region of the temporal arteries in older people. The finding of tender thickened temporal arteries suggests a diagnosis of temporal arteritis and blood should be taken for immediate measurement of blood viscosity or erythrocyte sedimentation rate (ESR). A presumptive diagnosis of this condition warrants immediate steroid administration and referral to a specialist physician.

A considerable number of patients are referred to the ENT clinic with the diagnosis of sinusitis when their only symptom is facial pain. It should be remembered that sinusitis is an infection of the sinuses which is usually associated with hyperaemia of the nasal mucosa and mucopurulent nasal discharge (see Chap. 4, section on The "Runny" Nose – Sinusitis).

The role of sinus X-rays is also discussed in Chap. 4 and it should be emphasised that a radiological report of "mucosal thickening" does not necessarily lay the blame for facial pain on the paranasal sinuses.

Trigeminal Neuralgia

This is an uncommon cause of facial pain. Paroxysmal bouts of pain occur in the distribution of one or more branches of the trigeminal nerve and are usually of short duration although they may be particularly severe. The aetiology of this disorder is unknown. The pain is almost always unilateral and there are often precipitating factors or "trigger" zones from where the initial stimulus may lead to a full-blown episode.

Treatment is with oral carbamazepine but it should be remembered that side-effects are common and regular blood counts are advisable. In severe cases the trigeminal ganglion can be anaesthetised or destroyed. There are some cases where an arterial loop is thought to press on the trigeminal ganglion in the posterior cranial fossa and this may be treated by interposition of muscle or fascia between these two structures.

Migraine

This subject is covered in detail in textbooks of Medicine and Neurology. This is an uncommon cause of facial pain seen in the ENT clinic.

Temporo-mandibular Joint Dysfunction

Several factors may lead to this condition including muscle spasm, malocclusion and jaw injuries. The affected joint is usually tender and although pain is often referred to the ipsilateral ear, the pain is commonly facial as well. These patients should be referred to their own dentist who will either deal with the problem or refer the patient to an oral surgeon if the underlying problem requires further specialist management.

Middle Turbinate Syndrome

A small number of patients complain of pain in the region of the ethmoid and frontal sinuses (Fig. 5.1). The General Practitioner's examination may reveal no abnormality and sinus X-rays may be unhelpful. However, anterior rhinoscopy may reveal a high deviation of the septum with the resulting deflection leading to contact between the septum and middle nasal turbinate. If the patient has pain when visiting the ENT clinic a cocaine test may be performed to assess whether or not middle turbinate syndrome is indeed the cause of the pain. A pledget of cocaine is inserted between the septum and the middle turbinate and the patient asked to wait for approximately 5 minutes. If the pain disappears (i.e. the cocaine test is positive) there may indeed be considerable benefit derived from amputating the middle turbinate and correcting the septal deviation.

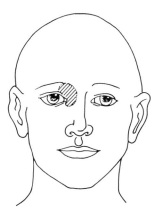

Fig 5.1. The site of facial pain in the "middle turbinate" syndrome.

Dental Neuralgia

Dental and periodontal sepsis should be sought and the teeth individually percussed to assess whether the teeth are the source of the pain. Dental referral is indicated if this is the case.

In general patients with facial pain are referred to ENT departments to exclude certain sites, such as the paranasal sinuses, as a cause of the pain. The ENT surgeon should routinely examine the entire head and neck after obtaining the appropriate history. Any treatable condition is then treated accordingly. However, if the site of origin of the pain is felt to arise in the teeth or temporomandibular joint, the patient will be referred to an oral surgeon. If a source is not found, a neurological opinion may be sought or referral to a pain clinic may be appropriate.

6 Facial Nerve Palsy

Facial nerve paralysis may arise from upper motor neurone problems such as those arising from a cerebrovascular accident, or the paralysis may be of lower motor neurone origin. Virtually all solitary facial nerve palsies seen in General Practice are of lower motor neurone origin. It should be remembered that the facial nerve makes a long journey from its origin in the pons, through the temporal bone, crossing the middle ear, traversing the mastoid bone and emerging at the stylomastoid foramen. It then enters the substance of the parotid gland before supplying the muscles of facial expression.

When a patient presents with unilateral facial weakness or complete paralysis, it is essential to test all the cranial nerves to establish whether this is a mononeuropathy or whether it forms part of a more widespread polyneuropathy. It is also crucial to examine the ipsilateral ear to ensure that a treatable cause (e.g. otitis media, cholesteatoma) is not being missed.

Bell's Palsy

This is the commonest cause of facial nerve palsy seen, the diagnosis being essentially one of exclusion. Its aetiology is unknown but many people think it is of viral origin. There is sometimes a history of a preceding upper respiratory tract infection which has given support to this theory.

If a diagnosis of Bell's palsy is made, the patient can be reassured that complete recovery is the most likely end result although this may take up to 6 months. Paralysis of the orbicularis oculi muscle may prevent adequate closure of the eye on that side with consequent drying of the eye. This may lead to soreness and ultimately corneal ulceration if the eye is not adequately protected. Artificial tears (e.g. hypromellose) should be prescribed and an eye pad worn if necessary. At night some form of eye ointment should be used to protect the cornea during sleep (e.g. 6% sulphacetamide or chloramphenicol). If it is thought that the cornea is at risk, then an ophthalmological opinion should be sought.

There is no evidence that any medication (including steroids) is of value or that physiotherapy has any influence on the eventual outcome or the speed of recovery. If there is any question of an otological disorder causing the palsy, then ENT referral is mandatory. Any facial nerve palsy that has not resolved or shown signs of resolution after 6 weeks should be referred to an ENT surgeon.

Facial Nerve Trauma

This may result from skull fracture involving the temporal bone or from facial lacerations. The facial nerve may also be injured during surgical procedures. These include operations on the middle ear and mastoid, or surgery of the parotid gland. Skull trauma of such severity as to cause a facial nerve palsy or a laceration of the facial nerve both require immediate specialist referral so that appropriate decisions can be made regarding the most suitable investigations, management and timing of repair of the nerve where indicated.

Parotid Tumours

Facial nerve palsy associated with a parotid tumour normally implies that the parotid lesion is malignant. However the commonest parotid tumours are benign pleomorphic adenomas and these do not as a rule cause facial nerve paralysis.

Treatment of a malignant tumour of the parotid gland may result in the facial nerve having to be divided. However, it may be possible to repair or graft the nerve at a later date. Alternatively, various re-animation procedures of the face may be performed to alleviate the unsightly appearance resulting from a facial nerve paralysis.

Tumours of the Facial (VII)
and Vestibulo-cochlear (VIII) Nerves

Facial nerve neuroma and "acoustic neuroma" are both rare but may result in a facial nerve palsy. A tumour of the facial nerve itself is an obvious reason for a facial nerve palsy. A tumour of the VIIIth cranial nerve may cause a facial nerve palsy due to the close proximity of the two nerves both in the cerebello-pontine angle and also in the internal auditory meatus.

Generalised Neurological Disorders

Facial nerve palsy may be a manifestation of many systemic neurological disorders such as neurofibromatosis, multiple sclerosis and sarcoidosis.

7 The Mouth and Throat

The Sore Mouth/Throat

Pain in the mouth and/or throat may be due to a variety of disorders. Pain in the mouth alone, e.g. the buccal mucosa and tongue, is usually due to a localised lesion which can be seen and/or palpated. Disease processes affecting the throat are only visible to the General Practitioner if they involve the tonsils or pharyngeal wall. Diseases occurring lower down, e.g. involving the epiglottis and larynx, require skill in the use of laryngeal mirrors.

Diffuse inflammation of the buccal mucosa may be due to vitamin deficiency disorders or may follow radiation treatment for head and neck malignancies. Treatment involves replacement therapy (e.g. vitamin B complex) in the former group and symptomatic relief in the latter (see Chap. 8). Avoidance of foods that are too hot or too cold and avoidance of salty or spicy foods lessens the discomfort but the patient often knows which foodstuffs to avoid from personal experience. It is important in all these conditions to be aware that the discomfort of drinking or eating may predispose to dehydration and this should be prevented. Diffuse inflammation of the oral and buccal mucosa associated with specific lesions of these surfaces may be due to a multitude of disorders which are listed in any authoritative textbook (see Appendix). The practitioner's duty is to assess the severity of the condition, to decide whether it is due to an infective agent or is part of a systemic disorder, or whether it is due to a local malignancy. The history is again crucial and the examination should be followed by microbiological swabs or biopsies depending on which is appropriate. Any failure of response to treatment warrants specialist referral. It should be emphasised that lesions in the mouth and on the tongue are often better assessed by palpation rather than by inspection alone. The lymphatic drainage areas in the neck should also be assessed as part of the examination.

Tonsillitis

This deserves special mention as recurrent tonsillitis is a very common disorder in General Practice and is probably the commonest condition referred to the ENT Department. In addition the indications for tonsillectomy are often controversial and difficult for the ENT surgeon to apply.

The specialist must rely heavily on the General Practitioner's referral letter as it is the family doctor who sees each attack of tonsillitis. The greatest difficulty lies in his assessment of those patients who have had recurrent "sore throats". It is essential to establish that these episodes have indeed been due to bacterial tonsillitis rather than to pharyngitis which is usually of viral origin. Once the diagnosis of recurrent tonsillitis has been made, the severity, duration and frequency of each episode must be assessed. At one end of the spectrum is the patient who has one attack per year which resolves rapidly on a course of antibiotics. Clearly this patient does not require tonsillectomy. At the other end of the spectrum is the patient who has several attacks per year that not only require antibiotic treatment but also cause the patient considerable debility and absence from work or school. This patient obviously needs a tonsillectomy. The difficulty lies with those patients that fall in between and here the decision will vary from one surgeon to another. Patients should be advised that tonsillectomy will prevent further attacks of tonsillitis but that "sore throats" may still occur later on. They should be warned that tonsillectomy is not a cure for viral or bacterial pharyngitis.

By far the commonest organism responsible for tonsillitis is the B-haemolytic streptococcus which remains sensitive to penicillin and so this is still the drug of choice unless there is a history of penicillin allergy. It is disturbing to see how many other antibiotics are used unnecessarily for this condition. In view of the erratic absorption of oral penicillin, it is imperative that therapeutic doses are prescribed and that their intake in relation to meals is adhered to (i.e. at least 30 minutes before food). The majority of cases of tonsillitis seen in the ENT clinic which have failed to respond to treatment persist as a result of inadequate dosage.

Tonsillitis is frequently a presenting feature of infectious mononucleosis caused by the Epstein–Barr virus. If this is suspected then other features of the disease should be sought. These include palatal purpura, marked localised lymphadenopathy which usually becomes more generalised along with hepato-splenomegaly. Haematological investigations reveal the presence of abnormal monocytes in the peripheral blood film and liver function tests are deranged to a variable degree. Treatment is mainly symptomatic (analgesia and antipyretics). The ampicillin group of drugs must be avoided because of the skin rash they produce in this disorder. There is a much slower resolution of the tonsillitis in this condition and the tonsils may be so enlarged as to cause upper airway obstruction. Such severe cases should be admitted to hospital.

Peritonsillar Abscess (Quinsy)

This is a collection of pus between the tonsil and its immediate lateral relation, the superior constrictor muscle of the pharynx. For unknown reasons this condition is almost unheard of in pre-pubertal children and has a peak incidence in adolescence and early adulthood. The patient has usually had tonsillitis for a week to 10 days when the abscess develops. There is general malaise, pyrexia, inability to eat or drink and dehydration frequently supervenes. On examination, there is marked trismus, halitosis and a large swelling pushes the tonsil and uvula across the midline. Treatment involves incision of the abscess and drainage of the pus under local anaesthetic, a procedure that brings rapid relief to the patient. This should be followed by high-dosage antibiotics (penicillin and metronidazole are the drugs of choice) and rehydration. Most of these patients require admission to hospital until they are able to drink adequately. Peritonsillar abscess used to be a rigid indication for subsequent tonsillectomy, but most surgeons would now only consider this if there is a history of recurrent tonsillitis or a previous quinsy.

The Lump in the Throat

This is a common presenting complaint in General Practice and is a common reason for referral to the ENT clinic. The majority of these patients, more frequently female, have no demonstrable cause for this symptom and they merely require reassurance that they do not have any major disease present. It is essential to exclude any serious disease process and it is also important that the patient can see that this has been done. A very small number of patients do indeed have a local lesion causing their symptoms. Some have gastro-oesophageal reflux as the cause of the problem which can be demonstrated radiologically or at upper GI endoscopy. In the majority of patients presenting with a lump in the throat, the aetiology is unknown. Whether this symptom is due to anxiety or cricopharyngeal muscle spasm (which may itself be due to anxiety) is open to debate. Nevertheless, following referral the ENT surgeon should take the appropriate history, examine the laryngopharynx and hypopharynx and order any further investigations where indicated. These may include a full blood count to exclude iron-deficiency anaemia (as in the Plummer–Vinson syndrome) and a barium swallow, specifically asking the radiologist to look for gastro-oesophageal reflux and also pharyngeal or upper oesophageal lesions. The results of these investigations seldom point to a specific aetiology and the origin of the "globus" syndrome remains unresolved.

If any local lesion is suspected either clinically or following radiological investigations, endoscopic examination should be performed. These patients are greatly relieved to know that there is nothing actually amiss and this in itself is usually curative. In those whose symptoms persist following negative investigations the possibility of a depressive illness should be considered and appropriate treatment commenced.

Hoarseness

This is both a symptom and a sign in which there is an alteration in the character of the voice. For practical purposes in General Practice, any alteration of the voice constitutes hoarseness and should alert the practitioner to the possible accompanying dangers of this symptom. There are many causes of hoarseness with certain conditions more common in each age group. Thus in babies, a hoarse voice or cry points to an inflammatory condition or congenital abnormality of the larynx. In children inflammatory conditions, congenital abnormalities or vocal nodules may be the causative factors. In adults, inflammatory conditions or neoplasms should be borne in mind.

Laryngitis

The majority of patients presenting to the General Practitioner with hoarseness are children and adults with laryngitis. This is usually a viral condition which generally accompanies an upper respiratory tract infection. It is aggravated by voice usage and smoking. Treatment involves voice rest, antibiotics if bacterial superinfection is suspected and methods of symptomatic relief such as steam inhalations and analgesics. Any patient with a hoarse voice that does not respond to treatment and fails to resolve within a finite period (6 weeks maximum) should be referred to a specialist for visualisation of the larynx. Hoarseness may be accompanied by upper airway obstruction if the causative disease process obstructs laryngeal airflow. The presence of such obstruction demands emergency treatment and immediate specialist referral.

Vocal Nodules (Singer's Nodules)

These occur as a result of voice abuse and may occur in children who shout excessively or in adults who abuse their voices in a variety of ways. People who work in noisy environments and have to shout above the level of the ambient noise are predisposed to the development of vocal nodules as are singers (trained and untrained). The nodules are not true neoplasms but represent localised areas of subepithelial oedema at the junction of the anterior and middle thirds of both vocal cords. Small nodules may respond to a course of speech therapy but larger nodules or the patient's inability to attend speech therapy usually indicate the need for surgical removal. After removal the patient should be advised by a speech therapist on the avoidance of voice abuse to minimise the likelihood of recurrence.

Croup and Epiglottitis

See section on The Obstructed Airway.

Carcinoma of the Larynx

Less than 5% of all laryngeal neoplasms are benign (polyps, papillomas etc.). Thus laryngeal carcinoma accounts for 95% of laryngeal tumours. Smoking and alcohol are the best-recognised associated or aetiological factors. Any patient whose hoarseness has not resolved spontaneously or with treatment after a period of 6 weeks should be considered to have a laryngeal carcinoma until proved otherwise. Any alteration in the mucous membrane lining of the true vocal cords will produce hoarseness. Therefore carcinoma of the true vocal cords (glottis) presents early due to an early change in the voice. Carcinomas of the subglottis and supraglottis usually present later as these areas have a larger space in which the tumours may expand and they therefore only present when they cause obstruction or they invade structures such as the vocal cords (causing hoarseness) or nerves (causing pain). The earlier the diagnosis is made the greater is the potential for cure, thus early referral of a suspected case of malignancy is mandatory. Early carcinoma of the larynx is usually treated by radiotherapy and cure is likely in most instances. Surgery is usually reserved for more extensive lesions or tumours that fail to respond to radiotherapy. Partial removal of the larynx may permit retention of voice-producing mechanisms but total laryngectomy necessitates the learning of new methods of voice production.

Vocal Cord Paralysis

The commonest cause of vocal cord paralysis is surgical trauma to the recurrent laryngeal nerve during neck operations, especially thyroid surgery. The paralysis may be merely a temporary one due to "bruising" of the nerve or the nerve may actually be severed. A small number of people have a congenital recurrent laryngeal nerve paralysis. A further group of patients suffer recurrent laryngeal nerve paralysis due to pressure on the nerve by disease processes in the left chest (only the left recurrent laryngeal nerve enters the chest). These include lung cancer, aortic aneurysm and left atrial hypertrophy. The right and/or left recurrent laryngeal nerves may be involved in malignant disease of the cervical lymph nodes or in anaplastic thyroid carcinoma.

The voice in unilateral vocal cord paralysis is usually "breathy" or weak until the uninvolved vocal cord compensates and moves further across the midline in phonation to "meet" the paralysed vocal cord. If the superior laryngeal nerve is also affected, there may be diminished sensation of the supraglottic larynx and this, combined with inadequate glottic closure, may lead to aspiration of saliva and food into the lower respiratory tract.

Bilateral simultaneous vocal cord palsy may be due to a viral neuropathy, bilateral recurrent laryngeal nerve damage or anaplastic thyroid carcinoma. These patients are not only hoarse but also usually have severe airway obstruction requiring a tracheostomy.

The Obstructed Airway

For the purposes of a book on ENT problems, only the "upper" airway is considered here. This includes the nose, nasopharynx, oropharynx, larynx and trachea as far as the carina or bifurcation. The symptoms and signs of upper airway obstruction vary according to the site of the obstruction and the rapidity of the onset.

The Nose

See Chap. 4, section on The Blocked Nose

Adenoids

Adenoids are a collection of lymphoid tissue situated on the posterior pharyngeal wall in the nasopharynx. Adenoids are largest in childhood and then undergo atrophy from puberty onwards. They may be so large as to cause significant airway obstruction. This condition may or may not be associated with hypertrophy of the tonsils. Children with enlarged adenoids often snore, are unable to breathe through their noses and so breathe through their mouths constantly. They may be irritable and tired during the day due to a disturbed sleep pattern at night. When the parents have observed the child sleeping, they may describe the signs of sleep apnoea. These are periods during sleep when there is temporary cessation of respiration. As a result of apnoea there is an accumulation of carbon dioxide and this provides the necessary stimulus for the respiratory centre to start breathing again. These spells are of short duration but are associated with significant hypoxia and disturbance of the sleep pattern. In its severest form sleep apnoea may lead to cardiac arrhythmias, pulmonary hypertension and death. These children require adenoidectomy, and tonsillectomy may also be required if both these areas are contributing to the problem.

Tonsils

Enlarged tonsils may also cause significant upper airway obstruction and the symptoms and signs are similar to those seen in patients with enlarged adenoids (see above). Additional features often mentioned by the parents are that these children are very noisy eaters and take a long time to eat their food. This occurs because the large obstructing tonsils make eating and breathing simultaneously a difficult and tiresome task. Obstruction of the upper airway by enlarged tonsils is a condition usually seen in children but it is occasionally seen in adults as well. Unilateral tonsillar enlargement should always arouse suspicion of malignant disease and specialist advice should be sought where doubt exists.

Snoring in children is almost always due to enlarged adenoids and/or tonsils. Snoring in adults may be due to enlarged tonsils but may also be due to nasal obstruction, e.g. a deviated septum or enlarged inferior turbinates. Some adults have rather lax pharyngeal and palatal musculature and when they sleep on their backs in particular, the flaccidity of these structures may cause them to prolapse into the upper airway. Snoring in these patients is a manifestation of an obstructed breathing pattern and this has on occasions led to marital difficulties. The problem of hypoxic episodes may also exist if the obstruction is severe. These patients are often overweight and somewhat plethoric! If the condition is severe, an operation called uvulopalatopharyngoplasty can be performed (see Glossary).

Larynx

Airway obstruction at the laryngeal level usually causes stridor, the noisy breathing associated with such obstruction. Disorders or lesions involving the vocal cords themselves will also cause hoarseness.

Croup

The commonest cause of upper airway obstruction in young infants is probably croup or laryngotracheobronchitis. This is usually a viral infection and the main area responsible for the severity of symptoms is that region immediately below the vocal cords (subglottis). This is the narrowest part of the upper airway, particularly in infants, and a small degree of mucosal swelling due to any inflammatory process causes a significant reduction in airflow. Children with croup require admission to hospital as a matter of urgency if there is any suggestion of airway obstruction, e.g. distress, restlessness, rib recession, cyanosis. In older children, the subglottis is larger and therefore significant airway obstruction occurs much less frequently. Treatment of croup includes humidification, nebulised adrenaline and airway intervention in the form of endotracheal intubation if critical obstruction threatens.

Epiglottitis

Although it is mainly the epiglottis that is involved in this disorder, all the supraglottic structures become oedematous and contribute to the airway obstruction. "Supraglottitis" would be a more accurate term. This condition is usually caused by *H. influenzae* and the differences between epiglottitis and croup, though not absolute, are summarised in Table 7.1.

The patient with epiglottitis is usually pyrexial, frightened and sitting upright in a position that helps splint the upper airway. Saliva drools from the mouth as swallowing is too painful. Breathing is shallow and stridor is a late and dangerous sign. The patient should be disturbed as little as possible as anything that increases respiratory rate and effort (e.g. crying, gasping, etc.) may precipitate complete airway obstruction. No attempt should be made to examine the pharynx with a tongue depressor as this may also precipitate total obstruction. It must be emphasised that the moment of total obstruction in epiglottitis is unpredictable and suspicion of the condition necessitates urgent admission to hospital so that airway intervention by (usually) endotracheal intubation can take place.

This condition has a significant mortality and management in hospital should be a team effort involving anaesthetists and ENT surgeons together. Epiglottitis is fortunately far less common than croup.

Table 7.1. The differences between croup and epiglottitis

	Croup	Epiglottitis
Age	Infants/toddlers	Older children/adults
Prevalence	Common	Rare
Aetiology	Usually viral	*H. influenzae*
Symptoms	Stridor	Fever, dysphagia
Associated URTI	Present	Absent
Preferred posture	None	Sitting
Progression	Slow	Rapid
Laryngeal oedema	Subglottic	Supraglottic
Airway occlusion	Predictable	Unpredictable
Artificial airway	Uncommon	Always
Mortality	Low	High

Tumours

Both benign and malignant tumours of the larynx may cause airway obstruction. These require specialist assessment involving indirect and direct laryngoscopy to decide on appropriate treatment. Emergency tracheostomy may be required. It should also be noted that patients undergoing outpatient radiotherapy for such tumours may develop significant laryngeal oedema during their course of treatment. These patients obviously require immediate ENT assessment and they may also require a tracheostomy until the oedema has settled.

Congenital Laryngeal Problems

The commonest congenital laryngeal disorder causing airway obstruction is laryngomalacia (synonym: congenital laryngeal stridor). This is a condition affecting infants from birth in which there is exaggerated flaccidity of the supraglottic laryngeal structures. It occurs with varying degrees of severity but is mild in most cases. There is variable stridor, made worse by increases in rate and effort of respiration and when the baby is lying on its back. These factors cause the supraglottic structures to prolapse into the glottic opening causing obstruction. The condition seldom requires treatment and it usually resolves spontaneously by about the age of 2 years. Although laryngomalacia is the commonest congenital disorder of the larynx, it is on the whole uncommon. Other disorders such as congenital subglottic stenosis usually only present when an inflammatory process causes increased mucosal oedema within the larynx.

The Neck Lump

The commonest cause of a lump in the neck is an enlarged lymph node. Such lymphadenopathy is in turn most commonly due to infection. Other causes of a lump in the neck include thyroid swellings, thyroglossal cysts and branchial cysts to name a few. The dilemmas facing most doctors regarding lumps in the neck are:

1. What structure are they?
2. If they are lymph nodes, what site are they draining?

Infective disorders can be treated with appropriate antibiotics and the lymphadenopathy will generally subside. Most children have palpable cervical lymph nodes and these should only arouse suspicion if they are longstanding, asymmetrical and significantly enlarged. What is meant by "significant" is a matter of clinical accumen and once again, any doubt warrants specialist referral.

The major area of controversy has been in the management of the malignant neck node. This issue has been hotly debated in the past and although there is general consensus now, certain cases are still mishandled with serious consequences for the patient's prognosis.

If a lymph node in the neck is thought to be malignant, and the neoplasia is not likely to be of thoracic or abdominal origin, i.e. the node is not in the supraclavicular fossa, an ENT surgeon should make a thorough search of the upper "aerodigestive" tract to find its origin. If no obvious tumour is seen, blind biopsies are taken of the nasopharynx, tonsil and the base of the tongue. The object of this seemingly circuitous route for arriving at a diagnosis is to prevent the spread of tumour from within the confines of the node to the tissues and skin of the neck. Only if the source of the primary disease is not found is the node excised in toto. Incisional biopsy (as opposed to excisional biopsy) will almost certainly spread the tumour beyond the confines of the lymph node.

Dysphagia

Dysphagia implies difficulty in swallowing. Pain on swallowing is known as odynophagia. Dysphagia may be functional, e.g. due to muscular incoordination of the pharynx and/or oesophagus, or due to organic causes.

A great deal may be learned from the patient's history. He should be asked to point to the apparent site of difficulty in swallowing and he should be closely questioned concerning symptoms of indigestion, heartburn and waterbrash. His problem may be progressive and it is important to establish whether he has difficulty swallowing both liquids and solids. Physical examination may establish systemic debility with weight loss but other signs are often lacking except where advanced carcinoma of the pharynx or oesophagus is associated with cervical lymphadenopathy.

The General Practitioner can initiate investigations by arranging for a full blood count and a barium swallow to be carried out. The radiologist may indicate that the patient's problem lies in the lower oesophagus or at the cardia when surgical specialist referral or a direct request for upper digestive end-oscopy will be indicated. If the disorder affects the pharynx or upper oeso-phagus then referral to an ENT surgeon is required. Further investigation will then include indirect laryngoscopy as an outpatient procedure and may be followed by pharyngo-oesophagoscopy for diagnostic and therapeutic purposes.

8 Prescribing in ENT

This is not a comprehensive formulary but a suggestion for simple, safe and inexpensive prescribing. It is a good idea to use as few products as are necessary and to get to know them well with regard to their efficacy and side-effects. Thus certain products which the reader may use regularly may not be mentioned in this section. However, it is important that the practitioner should be well versed in the use of whichever drugs he/she uses. If these are satisfactory with respect to both therapeutic value and lack of side-effects, then their use should be continued. It is also worth remembering that some preparations cost less if bought without an NHS prescription, e.g. nose drops, wax softeners etc.

The General Practitioner should also establish that his local pharmacist keeps the preparations he prescribes in stock. It is useful to know the comparative costs of these preparations and the shelf-life of the various topical preparations.

Topical Preparations

The Ear

There is no place for the random use of ear drops for "earache". Specific causes of earache should be treated appropriately (see below) but there is no indication for topical analgesic or anaesthetic ear drops.

Otitis Externa

Aural toilet is a prerequisite in this condition. This may be achieved by dry mopping in the general practice situation and this is made easier by the use of hydrogen peroxide (10 volumes) drops. The drops are applied immediately prior to dry mopping as they help loosen the epithelial debris in the external canal. Following adequate toilet, a variety of ear drops may then be applied. If topical hypersensitivity is thought to be a problem, drops which contain antibiotics should be avoided. In fact, otitis externa often fails to resolve following the use of antibiotic-containing drops or is exacerbated by their use. It is probably the steroid component of the drops that is the most active therapeutic ingredient and it may be worthwhile avoiding all topical antibiotics in this condition.

Suggested Preparations
- Glycerine and ichthammol drops
- Locorten-Vioform (clioquinol 1%; flumethasone 0.2%)
- Aluminium acetate 13%
- Betamethasone 0.1% (Betnesol)
- Clotrimazole 1% (Canesten) – if superimposed fungal infection is present (otomycosis).

These preparations should be applied three times a day.

Otitis Media

Topical preparations are only indicated if there has been a tympanic membrane perforation with resultant otorrhoea (i.e. perforated acute otitis media or chronic suppurative otitis media (see Chap. 2). Aural toilet should precede the administration of topical preparations. Again it is probably the steroid component of the drops that is the most active ingredient.

Suggested Preparations
- Sofradex (dexamethasone 0.05%; framycetin 0.5%; gramicidin 0.005%)
- Locorten-Vioform (clioquinol 1%; flumethasone 0.02%)
- Gentisone HC (gentamicin 0.3%; hydrocortisone 1%)

These preparations should all be applied three times a day

Wax

Wax can be softened prior to removal with a variety of preparations.

Suggested Preparations
- Arachis oil ear drops
- Sodium bicarbonate 5% ear drops
- Glycerol ear drops
- Olive oil

These drops should all be instilled three times a day until the wax is soft enough for removal.

The Nose

Decongestants

- Ephedrine 0.5% nose drops, applied three times a day.
- Xylometazoline 0.1% nose drops (0.05% paediatric), applied twice daily.

Both these preparations are extremely effective when used for the correct reasons (see Chap. 4, sections on Sinusitis and Allergic Rhinitis). Prolonged use may lead to rhinitis medicamentosa. They should therefore not be used for more than 2 weeks at a time.

Decrusting Agents

– Alkaline nasal douche (the patient can dissolve bicarbonate of soda in the palm of his hand and then sniff the solution up his nose).
– Glucose 25% in glycerin nose drops

Both these preparations should be used three times a day.

These preparations are useful in patients whose nasal cavities are prone to excessive crusting. Thus they are valuable following nasal surgery and in patients with bleeding disorders where crusting leads to epistaxis.

Allergic Rhinitis and Vasomotor Rhinitis

– Beclomethasone dipropionate (Beconase) nasal spray. This drug is extremely effective in allergic rhinitis. Regular use is crucial for successful treatment. It is also useful for the prevention of recurrence of nasal polyps following their surgical removal.
– Flunisolide nasal spray (Syntaris) (as above).
– Budesonide nasal spray (Rhinocort) (as above).
– Sodium cromoglycate nasal spray. The usefulness of this drug has been superseded by the above two preparations.
– Ipratropium bromide (Rinatec) anticholinergic nasal spray. Useful for watery rhinorrhoea.

Nasal Vestibulitis

This is a staphylococcal infection of the nasal vestibule. A course of systemic anti-staphylococcal antibiotics should be used in conjunction with either of the following topical agents:

– Chlorhexidine nasal cream 1%
– Chlorhexidine 0.1%; neomycin sulphate 0.5% (Naseptin)

These preparations may be applied to the vestibule (anterior skin-lined part of the nasal cavities) three times a day.

The Mouth and Throat

Symptomatic relief of the "sore mouth". These preparations are useful in patients who have diffuse mucosal inflammation of the lips and oral cavity:

– Hydrocortisone pellets (2.5 mg). These may be sucked four times a day

65

- Nystatin 100 000 units/ml. 1 ml is placed in the mouth four times a day
- Chlorhexidine mouth wash (Corsodyl). 10 ml mouth rinse two or three times daily
- Triamcinolone (Adcortyl) in Orabase. This paste may be applied to ulcerated areas or painful lips two to four times daily.

Treatment of Herpes Infections

Acyclovir may be used for the topical and systemic treatment of herpes infections. These include "cold sores", herpes zoster oticus (Ramsay–Hunt syndrome) and bullous myringitis.

Acyclovir cream may be used topically and treatment should commence as early as possible.

Acyclovir tablets are effective against herpes infections when commenced early in the course of the infection. This would be the preferred route of administration in herpes zoster oticus. The therapeutic value of both these preparations needs to be carefully weighed against their considerable cost.

Systemic Medication

Antibiotics

The principles of prescribing antibiotics apply as elsewhere in the body. The antibiotics should cover the most likely organism cultured from appropriate swabs; they should be administered in therapeutic doses and they should be administered for a suitable time period.

The list of all antibiotics available is too lengthy and inappropriate for a book of this nature. Where appropriate the drugs of choice are mentioned in the chapter concerned.

Antihistamines

These drugs have a limited role in seasonal allergic rhinitis. They are useful when the "season" begins. However, their sedative side-effects and their susceptibility to tachyphylaxis (rapid development of tolerance by the body) limit their usefulness to the short term. In addition topical steroid preparations such as beclomethasone are so effective and have so few side-effects that they are the preferred treatment in allergic rhinitis.

Decongestants

Pseudoephedrine hydrochloride (Sudafed) is the only pure systemic decongestant available. It is not as effective as the topical preparations and may cause significant hyperactivity in children.

Anti-vertigo Preparations

− Cinnarizine (Stugeron)
− Prochlorperazine (Stemetil)

Cinnarizine and prochlorperazine are useful for the nausea and vertigo of labyrinthine disorders. Both drugs are used in the treatment of Ménière's disease.

Prochlorperazine is a phenothiazine derivative and is used in the treatment of nausea and vomiting associated with labyrinthine disorders. The parenteral route would be the preferred route of administration in severe cases with excessive vomiting. A sublingual preparation (Buccastem) is also available.

Specific Treatment of Ménière's Disease

Betahistine dihydrochloride (Serc) is an orally effective treatment for Ménière's disease. It is thought to exert its effect by reducing endolymphatic pressure.

Glossary

What the specialist's reply means

This chapter defines what is meant by the terms used in the specialist's letter of reply to the referring practitioner. It is not intended to be a complete dictionary of all medical terms related to ENT, but is intended to explain terms which the ENT surgeon uses daily and which are not necessarily familiar to those in branches of medicine other than ENT.

A

Adenoidectomy removal of the adenoid pad by curettage.

Antrostomy intranasal. The creation of a new, large, gravity-dependent opening for the maxillary sinus into the nasal cavity. This is performed to bypass a blocked or malfunctioning natural ostium or to currette the sinus mucosa for diagnostic or therapeutic purposes.

Antrum washout irrigation of the maxillary sinus (antrum).

Atticotomy exploration of the attic (roof) of the middle ear. Attico-antrostomy is a surgical exploration of the attic and mastoid antrum simultaneously.

Axonotmesis a nerve injury in which individual axons are disrupted. Recovery is possible but there is often a residual deficit

C

Cacosmia the subjective perception of a bad smell, i.e. by the patient in his own nose.

Caldwell–Luc this is an operation in which the anterior wall of the maxillary antrum is opened via a sublabial approach.

Caloric tests tests during which water at 7° above and 7° below body temperature is irrigated into the external auditory meatus (EAM) to assess the vestibular mechanisms of the inner ear.

Canal paresis this implies that the vestibule of the ear or balance organ is hypofunctioning.

Choanae posterior openings of the nasal cavities into the nasopharynx.

Cholesteatoma see Chap. 2.

Commando procedure operation involving combined resection of half of the mandible, the floor of mouth on that side and radical neck dissection.

Croup laryngotracheobronchitis (see Chap. 7, section on The Obstructed Airway).

D

Dysphagia   difficulty in swallowing. *See also* Odynophagia, Globus syndrome.

Dysphonia   this usually implies a "weakness" of the voice as occurs in nerve lesions affecting phonation or in functional disorders. *See also* Hoarseness.

Dysphonia plicae ventricularis   a functional dysphonia in which the false vocal cords are used excessively in producing voice.

E

Endolymphatic hydrops   the pathophysiological process occurring in Ménière's disease.

Epiphora   excessive tear formation. This is usually due to obstruction of the nasolacrimal duct.

Exostosis   bony overgrowth occurring in the external auditory meatus (EAM)

F

Frontal sinus trephine   drainage procedure of the frontal sinus. This is performed via a skin incision above the medical canthus of the eye.

Fronto-ethmoidectomy   an operation performed via an internal and external approach in which both frontal and ethmoid sinuses are exenterated. A large opening is then made from the fronto-ethmoid complex into the nasal cavity to facilitate adequate drainage.

Furuncle   boil. Usually refers to a staphylococcal infection of a hair follicle in the external auditory meatus (EAM)

G

Globus syndrome   sensation of a lump in the throat.

Glomus tumour   tumour of chemoreceptor cells:
glomus tympanicum – tumour arising from tympanic plexus in middle ear.
glomus jugulare – tumour arising from region of jugular bulb.
glomus extravagale – tumour arising from ganglion nodosum of the vagus nerve in the neck.

Glottis   refers to the true vocal cords.

Glue ear   also known as secretory otitis media. The presence of a collection of fluid behind an intact tympanic membrane.

Grommets   small ventilation tubes placed in the tympanic membrane. Their implantation is usually performed under a short general anaesthetic.

H

Haemotympanum   the presence of blood behind an intact tympanic membrane.

Hallpike's test   a test for positional vertigo

Hoarseness   an alteration in the character of the voice. This usually implies a "rough" quality of the voice. *See also* Dysphonia.

Hypotympanum   see Fig. 1.9.

L

Labyrinth   term used to refer collectively to the vestibular and cochlear apparatus of the inner ear.

Labyrinthectomy surgical destruction of the labyrinth.

Labyrinthitis viral or bacterial infection of the labyrinth.

Laryngectomy operation for removal of the larynx. This may be total, requiring a permanent tracheostomy, or partial.

Little's area confluence of blood vessels at the anterior end of the nasal septum.

Ludwig's angina infection of the floor of the mouth associated with submental and submandibular swelling. The resultant oedema may be severe enough to cause upper airway obstruction.

M

Mastoidectomy an operation to clear out disease from the mastoid air cells. The operation may be performed via a post-aural or an endaural incision. The term radical when used in relation to mastoid surgery means that the posterior wall of the external canal has been removed and the middle ear and mastoid have been converted into one cavity. The meatus has usually been widened as part of the procedure and these features should be evident on examining the ear. A cortical mastoidectomy involves an exploration of the mastoid air cells but the posterior canal wall remains intact. The ear therefore appears normal on examination, save for the post-aural scar.

Mesotympanum see Fig. 1.9.

Middle-ear cleft usually refers to middle ear, mastoid and Eustachian tube together.

Myringitis inflammatory process of the tympanic membrane itself. The granular variety is more common (see Chap. 2). Bullous myringitis is less common.

Myringoplasty an operation to repair the tympanic membrane. This term is used interchangeably with type I tympanoplasty. The operation may be performed through the external auditory meatus (EAM) or via a post-aural incision.

Myringotomy an incision in the tympanic membrane. This is performed for the insertion of grommets or to release pus in severe, acute otitis media.

N

Nares openings of the nasal cavities – anterior and posterior.

Neck dissection synonyms: block dissection, radical neck dissection. An operation performed for the removal of metastatic carcinomatous lymph nodes in the neck. The operation also involves removal of the ipsilateral internal jugular vein and sternocleidomastoid muscle. The accessory nerve (XI) is usually sacrificed as well.

Neurapraxia a reversible block in nerve conduction. This is usually associated with minor injury to the nerve involved. *See also* Axonotmesis, Neurotemesis.

Neurotemesis injury resulting in complete division of a particular nerve. This injury is irreversible without some form of nerve anastomosis.

O

Odynophagia pain experienced while swallowing.

Oro-antral fistula an abnormal, epithelialised connection between the oral cavity and the maxillary antrum or sinus.

Ossiculoplasty operation involving reconstruction of the ossicular chain.
Ostium refers to the natural opening of a paranasal sinus.
Otomycosis fungal overgrowth in the external auditory meatus (EAM).
Otorrhoea discharge from the ear.
Ozaena atrophic rhinitis.

P

Pansinusitis sinusitis involving all the paranasal sinuses.
Paracusis a symptom describing the phenomenon of hearing better in the presence of ambient noise. This is characteristic of a conductive hearing loss.
Pars flaccida that part of the tympanic membrane covering the attic of the middle ear (see Fig. 1.9).
Pars tensa that part of the tympanic membrane covering the meso- and hypotympanum (see Fig. 1.9).
Perisinus abscess an abscess occurring in relation to the sigmoid sinus as an extension of mastoid disease.
Peritonsillar abscess an abscess occurring between the tonsil and the superior constrictor muscle of the pharynx (the immediate lateral relation of the tonsil). This is a complication of tonsillitis. Synonym: quinsy.
Presbycusis the hearing loss associated with the ageing process.
Pure-tone audiometry a test of hearing using pure tones delivered by an audiometer.

Q
Quinsy see Peritonsillar abscess.

R
Ranula mucus retention cyst in the floor of the mouth.
Reinke's oedema accumulation of subepithelial oedema fluid in the true vocal cords. This condition is usually associated with smoking and voice abuse. It causes hoarseness and is treated by stripping of the vocal cords followed by speech therapy and stopping smoking.
Rhinoplasty a cosmetic operation to alter the external appearance of the nose.
Rhinorrhoea discharge from the nose.
Rhinoscopy examination of the nose – anterior and posterior.
Rinne test test of hearing using tuning forks (see Chap. 2).

S
Saccus synonym: endolymphatic sac. A blind-ending sac of the endolymphatic compartment of the inner ear.
Saccus decompression a surgical procedure for severe Ménière's disease.
Septoplasty an operation to straighten a deviated nasal septum.
Septorhinoplasty an operation combining straightening of the nasal septum with cosmetic alteration of the external appearance of the nose.
Shrapnell's membrane same as Pars flaccida.
Sinus tympani a recess of the middle-ear cavity.
Speech audiometry a form of hearing test using spoken words. *See also* Pure-tone audiometry.

Stapedectomy an operation for otosclerosis in which the whole stapes was removed. The name has been retained but most surgeons now make a small hole in the stapes footplate through which an appropriate prosthesis can be inserted.

Stridor the noisy breathing associated with upper airway obstruction.

Submucous resection an operation to remove a deviated portion of the nasal septum.

Synkinesis unintended associated movements of facial muscles. This is usually a result of misdirected regenerating fibres following a facial nerve palsy.

T

Tegmen roof of middle ear (tegmen tympani) or of mastoid antrum (tegmen antri).

Tinnitus see Chap. 2, section on The Noisy Ear.

Tracheoplasty reconstruction of the trachea.

Tracheostomy an opening in the trachea situated on the anterior aspect of the neck. This may be a temporary measure to bypass an upper airway obstruction or it may be a permanent "end" tracheostomy following a laryngectomy.

Trismus inability to open the mouth due to muscle spasm.

Tympanoplasty an operation performed with the aims of repairing the tympanic membrane, restoring the middle-ear transformer mechanism and protecting the middle ear. The various types of tympanoplasty (I–V) refer to the final position of the repaired tympanic membrane in relation to the ossicular chain and medial wall of the middle ear. A "combined approach" tympanoplasty is a synchronous exploration of the middle ear and mastoid leaving the posterior canal wall intact. *See also* Radical mastoidectomy.

Tympanosclerosis plaques of calcified material in the substance of the tympanic membrane. It is usually the result of some form of "injury" either in the context of middle-ear disease or as a result of previous surgery to the tympanic membrane. It is fairly common after the insertion of grommets. It is seldom of any consequence

Tympanotomy an operation to inspect the middle-ear cavity.

U

Uvulopalatopharyngoplasty an operation performed in adults to alleviate severe snoring problems. The operation involves excision of redundant and lax tissue from the tonsillar pillars and the soft palate.

V

Vasomotor rhinitis see Chap. 4.

Ventricle (larynx) a recess of the larynx between the true vocal cords inferiorly and the false vocal cords superiorly.

Vestibule (inner ear) that part of the inner ear associated with maintenance of the body's equilibrium.

Vestibule (nasal) the anterior skin-lined part of the nasal cavity.

W

Weber test a test of hearing using tuning forks (see Chap. 2).

Appendix

Addresses of useful contact groups and institutions

Royal National Institute for the Deaf (RNID)

105 Gower Street, London WC1E 6AH
Telephone: 01-387 8033

Provides: Employment, training and education advisory service
  Hearing advisory service
  Information and publications
  Library
  Medical information and advice
  Speaker service
  Speech therapy advisory service
  Technical awareness service
  Telephone exchange for the deaf
  Television for the deaf fund
  British Tinnitus Association

City Lit Centre for the Deaf

Keeley House, Keeley Street, London WC2B 4BA
Telephone: 01-242 9872

Provides: Hearing therapists training centre
  Lipreading teachers courses
  Communication skills courses
  Teachers of signing courses
  Speech therapy for the deaf
  Lipreading courses

Link, The British Centre for Deafened People

19 Hartfield Road, Eastbourne BN21 1TD
Telephone: 0323-638230

Residential rehabilitation for those with acquired hearing loss with their families. Help in adjustment and adaptation.

Nuffield Hearing and Speech Centre

Gray's Inn Road, London WC1X 8DA
Telephone: 01-837 8855

Unit for parents and children – residential 1-week courses for parents and children with hearing losses.

National Deaf Children's Society (NDCS)

45 Hereford Road, London W2 5AH
Telephone: 01-229 9272

Run by parents of deaf children – aims to promote deaf awareness and give support to families of deaf children. Has local branches.

British Deaf Association (BDA)

38 Victoria Place, Carlisle CA1 1HV
Telephone: 0228-48844

Run by deaf people for deaf adults. Has local branches.

British Association of the Hard of Hearing (BAHOH)

7/11 Armstrong Road, London W3 7JL
Telephone: 01-743 1110

For adults with acquired hearing losses. Has local branches.

Breakthrough Trust Deaf–Hearing Integration

Selly Oak Colleges, Birmingham B29 6LE
Telephone: 021427 6447

For deaf and hearing people.

Provides: communication skills training and aims to promote deaf–hearing integration.

National Association of Deafened People

9 Went Hill Close, High Ackworth, Pontefract, Yorkshire WF7 7LP

Ménière's Group

c/o BAHOH, 7/11 Armstrong Road, London W3 7JL
Telephone: 01-743 1110

British Tinnitus Association

c/o RNID, 105 Gower Street, London WC1E 6AH
Telephone: 01-387 8033

National Association of Laryngectomee Clubs (NALC)

39 Ecclestone Square, London SW11 1PB
Telephone: 01-834 2857

For laryngectomees and their families. Has local branches.

Royal Association in Aid of the Deaf and Dumb

27 Old Oak Road, London W3
Telephone: 01-743 6187

Reference Texts

Scott-Brown's Otolaryngology, 5th edition
Editor: Alan G. Kerr
Butterworth, London

Tumors of the Head and Neck, 2nd edition
John G. Batsakis
Williams and Wilkins, Baltimore

Oxford Textbook of Medicine
Editors: D. J. Weatherall, J. G. G. Ledingham and D. A. Warrell
Oxford University Press, Oxford

Subject Index